CREEK RELIGION AND MEDICINE

by
JOHN R. SWANTON

INTRODUCTION TO THE BISON BOOKS EDITION BY
James T. Carson

UNIVERSITY OF NEBRASKA PRESS
LINCOLN AND LONDON

⊗

First Bison Books printing: 2000
Most recent printing indicated by the last digit below:
10   9   8   7   6   5   4   3   2   1

Library of Congress Cataloging-in-Publication Data
Swanton, John Reed, 1873–1958.
[Religious beliefs and medicinal practices of the Creek Indians]
Creek religion and medicine / by John R. Swanton; introduction to the
Bison Books edition by James T. Carson.—1st Bison Books
p. cm.
Originally published: Religious beliefs and medicinal practices of the
Creek Indians: Washington, D.C.: U.S. Gov. Print. Off., 1928, in series:
Smithsonian Institution. Bureau of American Ethnology. Annual report;
42d; 1924/1925
Includes bibliographical references and index.
ISBN 0-8032-9274-0 (pbk.: alk. paper)
1. Creek Indians—Religion. 2. Creek Indians—Medicine. 3. Creek
mythology. 4. Creek dance. I. Title.
E51 .U55 42d   2000
299'.753—dc21
00-021701

This Bison Books edition follows the original in beginning this manuscript, which was originally included in the *42d Annual Report of the
Bureau of American Ethnology*, on page 477; no material has been
omitted.

INTRODUCTION
James T. Carson

I read *Creek Religion and Medicine* as an undergraduate, well before I had ever heard of ethnohistory. Not until my doctoral studies some years later did I come across ethnohistory as a methodology for studying the Native American past. The timing was important not just for my own development as a scholar but for the evolution of the subject as a whole. In the study of the Native Southeast, there is no chicken-and-egg question to bedevil students and scholars. Swanton came first, ethnohistory came second, and the field has developed in such a way that what was written in the early decades of the twentieth century continues to shape scholarship as the new century begins.

John Swanton worked for the Smithsonian Institution's Bureau of American Ethnology for more than forty years. He searched archives for historical documents that shed light on indigenous cultures, and he spent a lot of time in the field speaking with Native informants about their beliefs and their memories of the past. Swanton published his findings in dozens of articles and several books on topics as wide ranging as language, religion, and folktales, and one would be hard pressed to name a more influential figure in the development of Native American history. This book was published originally in 1928 under the title "Religious Beliefs and Medical Practices of the Creek Indians" in the forty-second annual report of the Bureau of American Ethnology, and it has had an enormous impact on how historians have written about the Native South.

What makes the book important is Swanton's identification of basic underlying features of Native culture in written historical sources and in contemporaneous oral testimony. Besides the circles and crosses that cropped up regularly in Creek dances, ceremonies, and rituals, he also pointed out the enduring importance of fire to Creek conceptions of their universe. Fire lay at the center of Creek religion not just as an earthly representation of their greatest spirit but as an everyday manifestation of their relationship to their creator. Medicines and dances tied the people to the animals and plants that inhabited the world around them and offered them tools with which they could both combat diseases and other misfortunes and commemorate their triumphs.

For all his ability to comb archival sources and catalog cultural features, however, Swanton rarely engaged in overt analysis. The task of transforming his initial findings into an applicable body of theory about southeastern Indian culture fell to later generations of scholars. Angie Debo was one of the first historians to study the Creeks, and she relied on *Creek Religion and Medicine* to ground her study of their removal in the native culture.[1] More than thirty years later, in his important *Southeastern Indians* text, Charles Hudson crafted what has become the orthodox interpretation of not just Creek religion but southeastern cosmology as a whole by combining Swanton's work on Creek religion with his colleague James Mooney's observations of the faith of Eastern Cherokees. The diseases and cures Swanton uncovered also played an important part in Hudson's treatment of Native medicine.[2] J. Leitch Wright's study of the Native South, *The Only Land They Knew*, echoed Swanton. Like Hudson, Wright based his construction of Native cosmology on this volume.[3] Other scholars built on the cultural baseline established by Swanton and refined by Hudson and wrote specific studies of Creek society and culture. Michael D. Green, for example, used Swanton's elaborate discussion of the Green Corn Ceremony to anchor his study in a Creek conception of the world while Joel Martin's *Sacred Revolt* turned Swanton's work in new and controversial directions. In her study of Creek trade, Kathryn Holland Braund relied on Swanton to demonstrate the persistence of Creek religious thought in the face of colonial expansion.[4]

If Swanton's scholarship has shaped what historians have written about the Creeks and the Native South, his use of informants has had little influence on the same scholarship. The book is full of Creek informants from Alabama, Oklahoma, and Texas as well as members of other tribes, and they add an important dimension to the author's work. What criteria he used in gathering their testimony, however, is hard to say beyond the fact that he sought out old people who remembered their traditions and whom he deemed "intelligent." His use of their testimony is problematic because he attributed discrepancies between their memories and the historical record to local differences and to the vagaries of personality and memory.

As a student of culture, John Swanton was, in hindsight, a bit naive. Rather than accept that cultures change over time and that a culture could adopt alien influences without forsaking its own values and beliefs, Swanton searched the historical record for cultural features that he could match with his own informants' statements. In the process he worked backward and forward to fashion a Creek culture that was in his mind pristine. On this count he was explicit, and he refused to countenance any adaptation the Creeks made to Euroamerican cultures. Indeed, in one case he doubted certain Creek beliefs about the moon because they "smack[ed] of white acculturation."

By refusing to accord any importance to cultural exchange and change over time, Swanton misconstrued living Creek culture as irredeemably tainted. In the process he had to push aside such innovations as horse raising, cattle trading, and cotton cultivation without exploring the impact such material changes might have had on Creek medicine and religion. Moreover, his unwillingness to consider Christian influences on Creek religion as authentically Creek renders his assessment of historic and contemporaneous Creek religion ahistorical. Without looking at such important innovations, his portrayal of Creek culture stands as a testament to a futile search for what he called the "aboriginal character."

In the end, the reader may well ask that if Swanton's writing is so problematic, why read him at all? The most important reason is that Swanton's work lies at the heart of an interpretation of southeastern Native cultures that has dominated scholarship from the 1930s until the 1990s. Although Swanton's model of Creek culture has shaped the historiography, it would be worthwhile to reinvestigate it to decide whether or not circles, crosses, and so forth were in fact essential cultural building blocks. In his study of Cheyenne culture, for example, anthropologist John H. Moore took apart the ethnographic canon on which Cheyenne history had been based and presented an interpretation of their history that would have been otherwise unimaginable.[5] Is Swanton due for such a revision? Several important topics discussed in the book that never figured in the overall analysis certainly merit further study. How did gender figure into Creek cosmology? How did Creek men and women partition power and influence? And, perhaps most important of all, how did contact with Europeans and Americans affect Creeks' conception of themselves, the world, and their place in it? Anyone who wants to undertake such an important project has to begin with John R. Swanton's *Creek Religion and Medicine*.

NOTES

1. Angie Debo, *The Road to Disappearance: A History of the Creek Indians* (1941; repr. Norman: University of Oklahoma Press, 1989), 22–25.

2. Charles Hudson, *The Southeastern Indians* (Knoxville: University of Tennessee Press, 1976), 122–29, 340–42; and James Mooney, *History, Myths, and Sacred Formulas of the Cherokees* (Asheville NC: Bright Mountain Books, 1992).

3. J. Leitch Wright Jr., *The Only Land They Knew: American Indians in the Old South* (1981; repr. Lincoln: University of Nebraska Press, 1999), 19–20.

4. Michael D. Green, *The Politics of Indian Removal: Creek Government and Society in Crisis* (Lincoln: University of Nebraska Press, 1982), 15–16; Joel W. Martin, *Sacred Revolt: The Muskogees' Struggle for a New World* (Boston: Beacon Press, 1991); and Kathryn E. Holland Braund, *Deerskins & Duffels: The Creek Indian Trade with Anglo-America, 1685–1815* (Lincoln: University of Nebraska Press, 1993), 24.

5. John H. Moore, *The Cheyenne Nation* (Lincoln: University of Nebraska Press, 1987).

CONTENTS

ILLUSTRATIONS

PLATES

TEXT FIGURE

RELIGIOUS BELIEFS AND MEDICAL PRACTICES OF THE CREEK INDIANS

By John R. Swanton

GENERAL REMARKS

The southern Indians, like other peoples, dealt not only with their environment as it was but with their environment as they conceived it to be, and one of the most important branches of ethnology is that which concerns this latter concept. Unfortunately, at the present day comparatively little may be gathered regarding their attitude on the broader aspects of belief that is free from suspicion of white influence, while on the other hand no early traveler among the Indians was sufficiently interested in them and sufficiently sympathetic to obtain and transmit a correct account of it. The writer who most nearly filled these requirements was the trader Adair so often quoted in previous papers, but unfortunately his assistance on this particular side of aboriginal life is seriously injured by a prepossession that the Indians were descendants of "the Lost Ten Tribes of Israel," and he read this prepossession into all of the religious activities of the people observed by him. Particularly he concluded that the meaningless vocalic sounds used by his red friends in songs were so many forms of the name Jehovah and that their repetition was a conscious or subconscious adoration of the Hebrew deity. Nevertheless he was an acute and honest observer and faithful recorder of the things he actually heard and saw, so that it is usually possible to separate the facts from his deductions. With his help, the little that is furnished us by other writers, the information that I have myself been able to collect, and that obtainable from native myths and legends, the following outline of Creek religious beliefs has been put together.

THE COSMOS

Like all other primitive peoples, the southeastern Indians conceived of the earth as a flat plane overarched by a solid vault. To General Hitchcock Tukabahchee miko expressed the opinion that the world is square. Eakins, whose information comes principally from an Alabama Indian, says "they generally entertain the belief that the earth is a square figure, and entirely surrounded by water; and by going to the verge of the plain, they could step off."[1] And, in another

---

[1] Schoolcraft, Ind. Tribes, vol. I, p. 269.

place he observes "they believe the sky to be a material mass of some kind" and "that it is of a half-circular form, but that its truncations do not touch the earth." [2] The vault or sky was supposed to rise and fall upon the earth at intervals so that, by watching his opportunity, a person could pass under its edge. According to the same authority and my native informant, Jackson Lewis, the old people believed that the stars were stuck upon the under side of the sky, some of them, along with the sun and moon, revolving around the earth.[2] The constellation of the Great Dipper was called Pĭlo hagi, "the image of a canoe." The North Star was known as Kolasniegu, "the stationary star," the Morning Star as Hayàtitca, "bringer of daylight," and the Pleiades as Tukàbofkà.[3] A few other constellations and stars were also named.[4] Meteors were supposed to be "excrement cast upon the earth," and they mixed what they took for this with their medicines.[5]

Comets were thought to portend war. Some Natchez and Cherokee beliefs regarding them may here be inserted. In the language of the former a comet was called an'c tsū'nà, "chief of war"; it was believed to portend trouble for the whole people and a short life for the chief, or for the white men's President. The Cherokee are said to have called it " the big lion"; with them it was also a sign of war. The following story of a comet well illustrates the belief regarding such bodies and incidentally shows the small value of information when it comes from the superstitious. Watt Sam was my chief Natchez informant.

"Thirty one or thirty two years ago [from 1912] Watt Sam's grandmother, his brother, his sister, and Nancy Taylor, all of whom except the last are dead, had the following very singular experience. They lived close to Twin Springs, a mile to three-quarters of a mile north of where Watt Sam now lives. They were going to the cow lot a little after dark to turn the cows out when they heard a noise wï'dzidzidzidziti, and, looking up, they saw a snake chasing the moon. They were so frightened that they ran back to the house without letting the cows out. The snake chased the moon to a point half way between the zenith and the western horizon and stopped. Then it began moving its head back and forth, and they could see something green that looked like a snake's tongue. Its body extended half way across the sky, the tail being pointed toward the east. They could see something at the end of its tail which looked like rattles four feet long and a foot wide. The markings were like those of a diamond-backed rattlesnake. Its head was

---

[2] Schoolcraft, Ind. Tribes, vol. i, p. 269.

[3] Loughridge and Hodge have tcuk-lofka.—English and Muskokee Dictionary.

[4] From the Natchez I heard of a right-angled constellation which they called dü'gŭl gonŏ'gop, "the elbow stars." A tailed star, probably a meteor, was known as a "smoke star" (dü'gŭl bu'p'gubic).

[5] Schoolcraft, op. cit.

about four feet broad. They walked out into the yard and looked at it while the snake and moon remained still. Then they got frightened and went into the house, and the three children went to sleep. Their grandmother, however, was in distress, and did not know what to do. She went to the door every little while to look at the snake. By and by she got sleepy and fell into a doze. Then she awoke, went to the door, and looked again. She could not see it very plainly because it had grown dim. Then she went to bed again and slept a very long time, and when she looked once more she could see nothing of the snake and the moon had gone back to the east, to the place from which it had started. Watt was at Muskogee at that time with his mother. He has asked a number of people but never learned of anyone else who had seen this snake. At the time when this happened Creek Samy, an old Cherokee Indian, was out in the yard of his house with some other Indians playing cards. They did not see it either, but when they heard about it they said it was a lion that had flown across the sky. They claimed that a lion flew across the sky twenty or twenty-five years before that."

The galaxy was called poya fik-tcálk innini, "the spirits' road." [7] The aurora borealis was supposed to indicate changes in the weather "and always for the worse." [8]

The sun and moon were considered the abodes of powerful beings, or at least as connected with such beings; the former was evidently associated with the chief deity of the southern Indians to be considered below. Tukabahchee miko quoted the old people to the effect that the sun must be a great way off, "for if it came near it would burn everything up." When the sun or moon was eclipsed they said that a great toad (sábäkti) was about to swallow it, and in order to help drive it away they discharged their guns at it and shot at it with arrows until they "hit" it. Instead of a toad, Eakins was told of a "big dog," representing perhaps a distinctively Alabama idea. [9] My own informants asserted that the moon was not shot at when eclipsed, but this is an error. Tuggle adds his testimony to what has been given and on the occasion of a total eclipse of the moon, October 22, 1790, Caleb Swan says: "The Indians in all the surrounding [Creek] villages are yelling with fear, and firing guns in all directions. They have an opinion, on those occasions, that a frog is swallowing the moon; and make all their most hideous noises to frighten it away." [10] Adair tells us that the Indians of his acquaintance rejoiced at the appearance of the new moon[11] from which

[7] It was known to the Natchez as wácgup ū'ic, "dog trail," because it is supposed to have owed its origin to a dog who dragged a sack of flour along it, spilling the flour as he went, but this is also a Cherokee story (Mooney, Cherokee Myths, p. 259). A Cherokee informant added that his people sometimes said that the dog caused this whiteness from having gotten his paws into mortar.

[8] Eakins in Schoolcraft, Ind. Tribes, vol. I, p. 269.

[9] Schoolcraft, Ind. Tribes, vol. v, p. 269.

[10] Ibid. p. 254.

[11] Adair, Hist. Am. Inds., p. 76; see also Bartram, Travels, p. 495.

it is probable that they considered its waxing and waning either as a successive birth and death of entirely distinct bodies or as a wasting away and regrowth of one and the same. Another idea is suggested by Bartram in a footnote: "I have observed the young fellows very merry and jocose, at the appearance of the new moon, saying, how ashamed she looks under the veil, since sleeping with the sun these two or three nights, she is ashamed to show her face, &c." [12] In this connection might be quoted a speech which Pope states was delivered by an old doctor to the Coweta, Kasihta, and Broken Arrow people, after a very wet season, in which he says that the moon "had covered her face with a bear-skin" and concealed the stars with the tails of numerous beaver. [13] These declarations sound genuine though there is abundant evidence of "reading in" in parts of this speech. The moon was supposed to be inhabited by a man and a dog. Eakins, who makes this statement, also refers to a native idea that it is "a hot substance." [14] This smacks of white acculturation.

The rainbow was believed to be a great snake called Oskin-tatcà, "cutter off of the rain," its connection with clearing weather being well understood. "The old people knew," says Tuggle, "when they saw 'O-cee-kee-eer-tah-cher' that the rain would stop and that enough rain would never fall to drown the earth." He adds the important information that the rainbow cut off the rain by resting its two ends "on great springs of water." The Natchez call it et gwàht, "house neck." People spoke of running past it.

They believed in inhabited worlds—i. e., planes, both below and above that on which we dwell. Tuggle says:

"The earth is a very small island. . . . Indians live [on this and] also in the world under the earth. The third world is the sky world. The people of 'Esar-kee-tum-me-see' the Source of Life, the Life Controller, live in the sky world.

"Some say people (Indians) came down from the sky world, others say that they sprang from the earth, the soil, and hence the earth is man's mother and therefore sacred, and man cannot sell his own mother."

Tukabahchee miko told General Hitchcock that there are people living in the water and under the ground as well as upon the ground, and that the old people told him they had heard the drum [to accompany their dances]. [15] Eakins heard of a succession of inhabited planes underneath ours. [16] On the other hand no one seems to have mentioned a belief in more than one world above. This world above was thought to be the realm of departed souls as well as the dwelling place of many supernatural beings. The latter were considered benef-

[12] Bartram, Travels, p. 496.   [15] Hitchcock, Ms. notes.
[13] Pope, Tour, p. 61.   [16] Eakins in Schoolcraft, Ind. Tribes, vol. I, p. 269.
[14] Schoolcraft, op. cit.

icent and are said by Adair to have been called by the Chickasaw "Hottuk Ishtohoollo" (Hàták ishto holo, holy great men) or "Nana Ishtohoollo" (Nana ishto holo, holy great persons). With them he contrasts the "Hottuk ookproose (Hàták okpulosi), or "Nana ook-proose (Nana okpulosi)," "very bad men," or "very bad people," who, he says, were supposed to inhabit the dark regions of the west.[17] While Adair and other writers were likely to have interpreted Indian beliefs in the light of Christian teachings I believe this statement to be in the main correct. Swan mentions a good and bad region to which the souls of the dead go, and he says that a good spirit was over the one and an evil spirit—isti fàtcasigo, "person not good"— over the other.[18] This has a still stronger appearance of Christian influence, and, as I do not find the bad ruling spirit spoken of again by other writers, it may be doubted whether there was such a conception.

THE SUPERNATURAL BEINGS

Unlike the case of the bad spirit, a great good spirit ruling in the world above is mentioned by all early writers yet it is a question whether this was a native conception or not; the ease with which this spirit could be identified with the Christian deity and the fact that it was so identified in later times render the aboriginal character of the entire conception somewhat doubtful. The older Creeks assert that the name by which this being is now generally known, Hisagita imisi—now abbreviated to Hisagita misi—"the breath holder," is not the original term, but came in use after contact with white people. In explanation of the name it should be said that when an official was sent out in charge of a body of men at the time of the busk he was called an imisi, or "holder," because he held the body of men together. According to one informant the old name for God was Puyáfiktca lákàt, "the great spirit," but this man was a Baptist preacher and I believe the idea originated with the white people. Jackson Lewis, one of my best native informants, said that he recollected very well when the old people instead of calling the deity Isagita imisi used the term Ibofànaga (or Ibofànga), which means "the one above us." Nevertheless, as we find the name Hisagita imisi used by Adair[19] and all those of his contemporaries who enter deeply into the subject of Creek religion, we must assume that it is at least as ancient as the other term. What Lewis had in mind is probably indicated by another statement of his that in order not to use the term "Master of Breath," which was a very sacred name, directly, people often spoke of "the ones over and above us." The plural form in use here

---

[17] Adair, Hist. Am. Inds., p. 36.
[18] Schoolcraft, Ind. Tribes, vol. v, pp. 269–270; Hitchcock (Ms. notes) reports a similar belief.
[19] Adair, op. cit., p. 105.

suggests that originally the Creeks may have intended by the expression and the ceremonies directed toward the sky all of the spirits in the world above collectively. But, while there is probably some truth in this view, it seems pretty clear from the statements of early writers and mention of the "One Above" by the Chitimacha, Atakapa, and most of the other southeastern peoples, that they recognized a chief among these. Such a being was undoubtedly believed in by the Natchez, for their entire social system revolved about him, and there is every reason to think it was a prevailing southern belief. Bossu says that the Alabama called their supreme deity "Soulbiéche," [20] a word probably derived from solopi, "ghost," or "spirit," and ēsa, or īsa, "to live," to "dwell."

Adair gives the Chickasaw name of the supreme deity as "Loak-Ishtŏ-hoollo-Aba" [Luak Ishto Holo Àba], which appears to signify "the great holy fire above," and indicates his connection with the sun. Adair adds that he "resides as they think above the clouds, and on earth also with unpolluted people. He is with them the sole author of warmth, light, and of all animal and vegetable life." [21] His name at once suggests the Uwa' shiɫ ("Big fire") of the Natchez, which was their name for the sun, the highest object of their worship, or rather the abode of that highest object, and a connection between the Chickasaw and Natchez conceptions is thereby indicated. As to the regard in which the sun was held among the Creeks, Bartram says: "At the treaties they first puff or blow the smoke from the great pipe or calumet towards that luminary; they look up towards it with great reverence and earnestness when they confirm their talks or speeches in council, as a witness of their contracts; and also when they make their martial harangues and speeches at the head of their armies, when setting out, or making the onset, etc." [22] The idea involved, however, was probably much broader than that of the mere visible sun, because the latter was not considered a particularly imposing object. Adair says: "The American Indians do not believe the Sun to be any bigger than it appears to the naked eye. . . . Conversing with the Chikkàsah archi-magus, or high-priest, about the luminary, he told me, 'It might possibly be as broad and round as his winter-house; but he thought it could not well exceed it.'" [23] Compare, also, the statement of their beliefs which some Chickasaw are reported to have given to John Wesley: "We believe there are four Beloved Things above; the Clouds, the Sun, the clear Sky, and He that lives in the clear sky." [24]

Little else remains regarding the attributes of this deity which has not been entirely obscured by European beliefs. To show how far such beliefs had worked into the native conception, I will cite the

[20] Bossu, Nouv. Voy., vol. II, p. 48.
[21] Adair, op. cit., p. 19.
[22] Bartram in Trans. Am. Eth. Soc., vol. III, p. 26.
[23] Adair, op. cit., p. 19.
[24] Jones, Hist. of Savannah, p. 85.

following stories regarding the "Breath Holder" which were related to one of my oldest informants, a man born in Alabama before the migration to Oklahoma, by a very old Hitchiti Indian. This man said that a child was born in a certain country and a time came in the history of those people when children were to be killed. Rather than lose their child its parents put it into a basket, pitched it with gum, and set it afloat upon the water. Afterwards it was seen by the king, who told an attendant to bring it in, and he did so. Fascinated by its beauty he adopted it and reared it. One day after he grew up this child was walking along and saw a man planting seed. He asked him what it was and the man answered "I am planting stones." Later he went to this place again, dug into the earth, and found a great many stones there. Another time when he met this man the latter had some white corn flour. He threw a handful of this into the air and it turned into white water herons found along streams, the feathers of which were used in the Creek peace dance. The old man said that the man who did this was Christ and added that "a darn Frenchman came along and killed him." The myth of seed turning into stones is recorded in various versions by Dähnhardt, in his Natursagen, vol. II, p. 95, under the heading Die Verwandlung des Saatfeld. The other is a well-known episode in apocryphal church history. The first part of the narrative is of course taken from the story of Moses.

One further point regarding this spirit deserves notice, as it is certainly not European in origin, and that is his connection, in the minds of the Indians, with the sacred fire as several times mentioned by Adair. In one place he says, "they worship God, in a smoke and cloud, believing him to reside above the clouds, and in the element of the, supposed, holy annual fire." [25] Further on he goes into this more at length, as follows:

"Though they believe the upper heavens to be inhabited by Ishtohoollo Aba, and a great multitude of inferior good spirits; yet they are firmly persuaded that the divine omnipresent Spirit of fire and light resides on the earth, in their annual sacred fire while it is unpolluted; and that he kindly accepts their lawful offerings, if their own conduct is agreeable to the old divine law, which was delivered to their forefathers." [26]

Again, he quotes a Chickasaw seer to the effect that "he very well knew, the giver of virtue to nature resided on earth in the unpolluted holy fire, and likewise above the clouds and the sun, in the shape of a fine fiery substance, attended by a great many beloved people." [27] Adair backs these statements up with the following incident, which is of more importance than his bare assertion, and especially in this connection, as it is from the Creeks instead of the Chickasaw:

---

[25] Adair, Hist. Am. Inds., p. 35.   [26] Ibid, p. 116.   [27] Ibid., pp. 92–93.

"In the year 1748, when I was at the Koosah on my way to the Chikkasah country, I had a conversation on this subject, with several of the more intelligent of the Muskohge traders. One of them told me, that just before, while he and several others were drinking spirituous liquors with the Indians, one of the warriors having drank to excess, reeled into the fire, and burned himself very much. He roared, foamed, and spoke the worst things against God, that their language could express. He upbraided him with ingratitude, for having treated him so barbarously in return for his religious offerings, affirming he had always sacrificed to him the first young buck he killed in the new year; as in a constant manner he offered him when at home, some of the fattest of the meat, even when he was at short allowance, on purpose that he might shine upon him as a kind God. And he added, 'now you have proved as an evil spirit, by biting me so severely who was your constant devotee, and are a kind God to those accursed nothings [i. e., the white people], who are laughing at you as a rogue, and at me as a fool, I assure you, I shall renounce you from this time forward, and instead of making you look merry with fat meat, you shall appear sad with water, for spoiling the old beloved speech. I am a beloved warrior, and consequently I scorn to lie; you shall therefore immediately fly up above the clouds, . . .'" [28]

In still another place he says: "The Muskogee call the fire their grandfather—and the supreme Father of mankind Esakata-Emishe 'the breath master,' as it is commonly explained." [29] Fire is called "grandfather" to the present day.[30]

After describing the method of deadening trees and clearing fields among the southern Indians, Adair goes on thus:

"With these trees they always kept up their annual holy fire; and they reckon it unlawful, and productive of many temporal evils, to extinguish even the culinary fire with water. In the time of a storm, when I have done it, the kindly women were in pain for me, through fear of the ill consequences attending so criminal an act. I never saw them to damp the fire, only when they hung up a brand in the appointed place, with a twisted grape-vine, as a threatening symbol of torture and death to the enemy; or when their kinsman dies. In the last case, a father or brother of the deceased, takes a firebrand, and brandishing it two or three times round his head, with lamenting words, he with his right hand dips it into the water, and lets it sink down." [31]

All of the facts brought out must mean that an actual connection was supposed to exist between the sun and the busk fire and thus between the celestial deity behind the sun and this fire, and, as Adair himself points out elsewhere, that the renewal of the fire was an actual renewed presence of the deity among them, the old fire having

[28] Adair, Hist. Am. Inds., p. 116.
[29] Ibid., p. 105.
[30] Cf. Bartram in Trans. Am. Eth. Soc., vol. III, p. 26.
[31] Adair, op. cit., p. 405.

become polluted by long separation from its source.[32]   It is unfortunate that we have no further information on this important point.

Swan, the only writer who has much to say of a great evil spirit, remarks that "they have an opinion that droughts, floods, and famines, and their miscarriages in war, are produced by the agency of the bad spirit. But of these things, they appear to have confused and irregular ideas, and some sceptical opinions." [33]   I have already expressed doubts about the primitive character of the bad spirit but it is possible that a kind of dualism based on the opposing activities of the good and bad spirits collectively may have grown up.

Yahola and Hayū′ya were two important male deities supposed to reside together in the air without any other companionship. When novices were being instructed regarding the sacred medical formulæ and other mysteries in a way to be described presently the teacher sang songs in which the names of these two beings were mentioned very often. From the general drift of these songs it would appear that the two beings were perfect, clean, undefiled, and were in this manner implored to act as guardians and good geniuses of the pupils. To Jackson Lewis, to whom I am indebted for all of this important information, these beings seemed to endow one with strength, physical activity, and clearness of vision and thought. Yahola was also sometimes appealed to in sickness. If a person was shot and appeared to be dying some ginseng would be cut up and placed in a cup of water and a song sung over it containing the name of Yahola and appealing to his aid in this great emergency. Then the drink would be administered to the sufferer and by doing so it was thought that his life could be prolonged until a more thorough treatment could be undertaken. Also in cases of difficult childbirth the doctor would make medicine and over it utter an appeal to Yahola. "And," concluded Lewis, "this is the real Yahola, though you will find persons so named who do not know what the word means." This word was, in fact, employed in numerous war titles, and a cry called "the Yahola cry" and supposed to resemble the call of the deity himself, was uttered when black drink was taken, and on some other occasions during the annual busk. The name Hayū′ya gives us a clew to the four "Hi-you-yul-gee" from the four corners of the world who brought fire to the ancestors of the Creeks.

The being who produced thunder and lightning is identified by Adair with the supreme deity, for in one place he calls the latter "Ishtohoollo Aba Eloa" (the big holy one above who thunders).[34] He tries to represent what he conceives to be the native idea when he says that the divine power of distributing rain at his pleasure

[32] Adair, Hist. Am. Inds., pp. 105, 107.
[33] Swan in Schoolcraft, Ind. Tribes, vol. v, p. 270.
[34] Adair, op. cit., pp. 93–94.

"belonged only to the great beloved thundering Chieftain, who dwells far above the clouds, in the new year's unpolluted holy fire." [35] We are here reminded of a doctor encountered by Pope, who spoke of "the great God of Thunder and Lightning and of Rain." [36] The real native idea seems to be set forth, however, in the following quotation:

"The Indians call the lightning and thunder, *Eloha* [Hiloha, is thunder] and its rumbling noise, *Rowah*, . . . and the Indians believe . . . that *Minggo Ishto Eloha Alkaiasto*, 'the great chieftain of the thunder, is very cross, or angry when it thunders' and I have heard them say, when it rained, thundered, and blew sharp, for a considerable time, that the beloved, or holy people, were at war above the clouds. And they believe that the war at such times, is moderate, or hot, in proportion to the noise and violence of the storm.

"I have seen them in these storms, fire off their guns, pointed toward the sky; some in contempt of heaven, and others through religion—the former, to shew that they were warriors, and not afraid to die in any shape; much less afraid of that threatening troublesome noise and the latter, because their hearts directed them to assist *Ishtohoollo Eloha*." [37]

Here it is said that the cause of the thunder and lightning was warfare between many celestial beings, not the prerogative of a single one.

Jackson Lewis stated that it used to be said that the thunder was a person who possessed missiles (lĭ, the word employed here, may mean an arrow, a bullet, a sting, or a thunderbolt) and would dart them out toward the earth with great noise. There is also, they said, a long snake that rises out of the water and can produce the same kinds of noises as the thunder man, but the noises of the former are accompanied by blue lightning and are without a bolt. These two sometimes amuse each other, the thunder man making noises and throwing his bolts down while the thunder snake thunders back and shows the blue lightning. The snake is sometimes in the ground or under a rock out of sight when this happens, and the thunder man throws his bolts into the trees or rocks near by. It has been thought by some that the thunder man kills the snake with his bolts. Lewis claimed to have seen thunderbolts (tinitki inli) which looked like crystals, or at least had similar facets. Sometimes they are found where a tree has been shivered by lightning and sometimes in the water, but if one puts his hand into the water to get them the hand will become paralyzed. They are of the colors red, yellow, white, and blue, [38] and thus seem to resemble the sabīa to be described presently, but they were not identified with these.

---

[35] Adair, Hist. Am. Inds., p. 92.
[36] Pope, Tour, p. 60.
[37] Adair, op. cit., p. 65.
[38] In one place I have noted the colors as "blue, black, red, and white."

It is interesting to compare with this the notes on the subject by Tuggle, written at a much earlier period:

"The Muskogee say of lightning that a little man rides a yellow horse, and when he shoots his arrows, it thunders. Sometimes he shoots at a tree.

"When lightning—'Ah-tee-ya-hal-tee' (Atoyahàti)—strikes a tree and slightly injures it, some say this is caused by the terrapin. When the tree is torn to pieces, this is caused by the big noise (thunder)."

Tuggle recorded the following regarding the wind:

"The Wind was very destructive. The people wanted him to go away.

"The Wind said: 'I am going away to the other end of the world. I will sometimes send some of my servants back to visit you. Some will be soft and gentle, some will be rough and loud. When the end comes, the last day, I will come with great power and will sweep all to one place from the four corners of the earth.'

"So the Wind went away."

Reference to the earth as an island has already been quoted. Further light on the native conception of it may be gained from the several creation stories, which are in fact stories of how the present order of things was instituted out of a previous order of things of an analogous nature. I have been told that there was once a long myth of this kind, most of which has been lost. The following fragments will, however, present the native idea in general outlines very well. The creation story and the flood story are so mingled that it will be well to include both.

The agent Eakins, who obtained most of his information from an Alabama Indian, says on this point:

"They believe that before the Creation there existed a great body of water. Two pigeons were sent forth in search of land, and found excrements of the earth-worm; but on going forth the second time, they procured a blade of grass, after which, the waters subsided, and the land appeared."[39]

Speck secured the following myth from a Tuskegee medicine maker:

"The time was, in the beginning, when the earth was overflowed with water. There was no earth, no beast of the earth, no human being. They held a council to know which would be best, to have some land or to have all water. When the council had met, some said, 'Let us have land, so that we can get food,' because they would starve to death. But others said, 'Let us have all water,' because they wanted it that way.

"So they appointed Eagle as chief. He was told to decide one way or another. Then he decided. He decided for land. So they

---

[39] Schoolcraft, Ind. Tribes, vol. I, p. 266.

looked around for some one whom they could send out to get land. The first one to propose himself was Dove, who thought that he could do it. Accordingly they sent him. He was given four days in which to perform his task. Now, when Dove came back on the fourth day, he said that he could find no land. They concluded to try another plan. Then they obtained the services of Crawfish (sákdju). He went down through the water into the ground beneath, and he too was gone four days. On the fourth morning he rose and appeared on the surface of the waters. In his claws they saw that he held some dirt. He had at last secured the land. Then they took the earth from his claws and made a ball of it. When this was completed they handed it over to the chief, Eagle, who took it and went out from their presence with it. When he came back to the council, he told them that there was land, an island. So all the beasts went in the direction pointed out, and found that there was land there as Eagle had said. But what they found was very small. They lived there until the water receded from this earth. Then the land all joined into one." [40]

According to one of the fragments collected by myself, water covered everything in the beginning and no living beings existed except two red-headed woodpeckers, which hung to the clouds, with their tails awash in the waters.[41] When the water went down it left marks on their tails which remain to-day. It also left a muddy island, and on this seven persons were created, apparently by The One Above. By extending their thoughts these seven persons extended the boundaries of this island until it took on the dimensions of the present dry land. This fragment was from Tâl mutcási, late medicine maker of the Fish Pond and Ásilanabi towns. Big Jack, a leading repository of native lore among the Hilibi, said that anciently there was a flood of waters, upon which floated a canoe in which were some human beings and animals of all kinds. The opossum hung to the side of the canoe with its tail in the water, and that is how it happens to have a tail practically devoid of hair at the present time.[42] The red-headed woodpecker hung to the sky and the tip of his tail was discolored permanently. Afterwards the creatures wanted to get some earth. First the earthworm started down after it, but the fishes seized him and ate him up. Next the crawfish started down, but he did not come up again. Finally the dove flew away and brought earth from beyond the horizon, and from this the dry land of to-day was formed.

[40] Memoirs Am. Anth. Asso , vol. II, pt. 2, pp. 145–146.
[41] According to Tuggle they were sitting on the side of the ark, a later Christian adaptation. While Tuggle calls this bird "Phe-tuk-kee" (fituki), the yellow-hammer, my Alabama informants considered t was a bird a little larger than the common red-headed woodpecker (waháwágwá), called in their language itka.

This last story and the one obtained by Doctor Speck are interesting because they combine the peculiar Southeastern tale in which a bird brings the first land with the well-known quest for earth beneath the waters, a story found over the whole of the eastern part of North America.

According to the idea of the southern Indians, something of the supernatural attached to every created thing, every animal, plant, stone, stick, body of water, geographical feature, and even to objects which man himself had made. While these things did, indeed, have certain characteristic appearances and activities which were "natural"—that is, the things normally expected from them—they owed these to a certain impression made upon them in the beginning of things, or at least at some time in the distant past, and it was not to be assumed that they were all the powers which such beings and objects—or, assuming the Indian point of view, we might say simply beings—possessed. The expected might give way at any moment to the unexpected. In such cases the thing itself might exert power in its own right or it might be a medium of power from another being. It might manifest this power at one particular time to one particular person, it might have the faculty of exerting its power constantly, or its power might be brought out from it by the observance of certain regulations. In such cases the response might be an infallible result of performing the regulations, or the charm might be capable of exercising a modicum of volition.

An ability to talk on occasion was attributed to animals. Once a prophet heard an owl and a dog talking to each other. The owl said, "People must be afraid of me." The dog answered, "No, but if there is a big stick lying across the road they will be afraid of that." "Would they be afraid of a bush?" inquired the owl. "They would not be afraid of that; they would go around it." "But would they not be afraid if I should get on top of the bush?" "If you do it, they will kill you." They disputed about this for some time and at last the owl perched on a bush in the middle of the road to try and scare passers-by, but in vain.

The beings most important in the lives of the Indians or those which, for any reason, were most conspicuous were of course the ones which attracted the most regard from them, were oftenest referred to in their stories, and were made the occasion of something approaching a cult. Still this statement needs modification, since some of their conceptions were the result of evolution, and can not be said to have been due to any apparently greater significance of the objects or creatures in the lives of the present-day Indians. It is even uncertain that they ever were of cardinal significance; some chance association, or the influence of foreign peoples, may have given them their superior position. It should be added that some of the beings by which they believed themselves to be surrounded were purely imaginary. Their attitude toward these was theoretically the same as that toward the common creatures, but as they were not of every-day experience, the supposed encounters with them were of course always believed to have supernatural significance.

According to both the early writers and the present day Indians, in ancient times the Indians would not willingly kill a wolf or a rattlesnake. I was told that not many stories were related about the former because it was considered the friend of the red men and they were afraid it would injure them.

Not many stories were told about snakes for fear of receiving injury, and Bartram says that the Indians whom he met would not willingly kill any sort of snake, believing that if they did so the spirit of the snake would excite or influence his living kindred or relatives to revenge the injury done to him when alive.[44] Upon one occasion he killed a rattlesnake that had driven some Seminole from their camp, whereupon several of them came to him and performed a kind of ceremonial dry scratching upon him. This was evidently in order to make the relatives of the snake believe that the injury had been atoned for.[45] Adair records that misfortune was predicted by a Chickasaw doctor because he (Adair) had killed one of these reptiles.[46]

A great deal was made of "masters of waters," water creatures such as the beaver, otter, and water snake. They are often associated together in the linking of clans. When I was in Oklahoma during a very dry season, which had been preceded by two or three very dry seasons, some of the Indians said that this was due to the fact that since the coming of the whites the masters of waters, who anciently protected the earth from dryness, had lost control.

Just as we find on the north Pacific coast and elsewhere that the supernatural beings live when at home like men on earth, we hear in Creek stories of animal towns scattered about like those of the Indians, each with its square ground, though of course there are always supernatural accompaniments, and curious features reminding one of the animals which live there. The following story gives an experience with the under water people.

A man who was at some distance from his town fasting in order to obtain medicine was once out after wood, and saw a man up the creek from him, whom he presently met and conversed with. When he got back, he picked up his kettle and started after water, but, on reaching the branch, he threw his kettle into it. Then he stripped off

---

[44] Bartram, Travels, p. 261, note.
[45] Ibid., pp. 258–261.
[46] Adair, Hist. Am. Inds., pp. 272–273.

his shirt and dived under water after it. Two little snakes then took hold of him and guided him along, making a way for him so that he could breathe exactly as if he were on land. By and by they came to a place like a Creek square ground, but the beds were all made of snakes plaited together, and there was a big turtle in front for a footstool. Then the old snakes said "Why did you bring that person here?" But as long as they had done so, the old people told him to sit down. When he tried to step on the turtle, however, it raised up, and it did this three times. The fourth time it stopped and he stepped on its back. When he was about to sit down the snakes began crawling, but at the fourth attempt they also stopped and he seated himself. Then they asked him if he wanted a feather which was fixed in the roof above his head, and he said "Yes," but, when he tried to seize it, it flew up out of reach. At the fourth attempt he got it. Again they said to him, "Do you want that hatchet?" "Maybe I do," he answered. This also rose out of his reach three times and the fourth time he got it. "If you are a man," they said, "let us see you strike off the head of that turtle." So he got off of the turtle's back, aimed a blow at its neck, and, zip! off flew its head while its blood spattered round about. "This will do for you," they said, and they gave him all sorts of instructions as to how he could visit them. From that time on he went back to see them frequently, but presently he began violating their instructions, and they in turn began to dash water on him, so that at last he could not reach them. The man's name was "Horned" (Yábi odjà). He used to dive under water and return about noon with a string of turtles tied together with hickory bark. There was a whirlpool under some rocks in the South Canadian below the standing rock near the mouth of the North Canadian, and there he said he saw some creatures that looked like dogs and he thought that they might be dangerous, but he said that they did him no harm. One day, however, he got drunk and was found dead on the bluff just above that place.

Another boy, a grandson of the preceding, was able to stay under water so long that his companions thought he was drowned. But one time he saw something that scared him, and afterward he remained on shore. He said that the place to which he went was like an open space. It was thought that his grandfather must have taught him how to stay under water, as he would come out in the same way carrying a string of turtles tied together with hickory bark.

My informant affirms that these are true stories, and that an old Indian named Judge Nokosi with whom he was acquainted knew "Horned" personally. "Horned" was a Tukabahchee; the grandson, a Łaplåko.

A similar experience is related thus. It shows how a supernatural object was obtained for the inside of the "chief ball" used in the ball game.

An old Alabama doctor living in Oklahoma told a certain man to go into a creek to get part of the nest of a corduroy snake (tie snake) from a cave there, and he gave him a magic cane with which to quiet the serpents. The man went to the water, but, when he saw the snakes, he was afraid and went back. Then the doctor gave the cane to another man. This person went to the creek and began walking into the water, when it was just as if he were walking on dry ground. He saw the cavern with the snakes lying all about. Then he touched them with his cane and they did not hurt him. So he got a little of the nest of the snakes and brought it back, and that was what they put into the center of the ball with which they played.

According to one of my informants the "tie snake" referred to in this story was a long slender snake which made progress by a succession of jumps or flips and was so powerful that it could carry a full-grown horse along with it. Upon one occasion such a snake seized a horse near Wetumka, Okla., and was carrying it along to its den in this manner when the horse in its struggles kicked the snake on the head and killed it. Jackson Lewis, however, gave a somewhat different account of this snake, which I quote along with a story regarding it said by him to belong to very recent times.

The "tie snake" is an inch and a half in diameter and short, but it is very strong. It is white under the throat, but black over the rest of the body, and its head is crooked over like the beak of a hawk. It lives in deep water, usually in small deep water holes from which it makes excursions into the woods, drawing its prey down into the water to its den. There are many tales told of this tie snake, of which the following is a specimen.

A Creek Indian named Ogue hili ĭmăla, now dead, who used to live about 3 miles from Eufaula, told this to Lewis as a personal experience. He once owned a mare which had a colt. Having missed his mare from the range, he hunted for some time, and finally found her by means of the colt, which he saw running about but always returning to a certain spot. Finally he went to this place and saw that a large tree had been uprooted there, leaving quite a hole where its roots had been—a hole partially filled with water. There he found his mare with her hind quarters under water and her head and shoulders out. As he could not get her out alone he gathered his neighbors together and they went to the place with ropes which they tied about the mare's body and pulled on all together in order to draw her out. But their efforts were at first fruitless. Making a supreme effort, however, they were successful, whereupon the water seemed to flow in from all quarters and fill up the hole. The mare was not much hurt, and they took her away and cared for her until she recovered. Her hind quarters were at first numbed, however, and upon them was a spot about an inch and a half across from which the hair had been rubbed. The skin there became black and finally scaled off. When the hair came out again it was black and the animal was quite a curiosity on account of the black ring. Everybody, including Lewis, felt perfectly satisfied that a tie snake had caught this mare and dragged her into the water hole.

This snake is said to have originated from a transformed human being. Two hunters were out together and in a certain place they found two eggs. One of them was suspicious of these but the other was a rash, heedless youth, and he ate them. That night he began to feel strange and his companion observed that he was changing his shape. This change went on until he became a great serpent which continued to live in a water hole near by. Afterwards his mother came to see him and he recognized her but returned again into the water.[47]

In the Tuggle collection there is a note of another snake, known as "the sharp breasted snake," [48] but I obtained a very much better account of this creature from Jackson Lewis. The two accounts disagree in no particular. Lewis's account is as follows:

The sharp-breasted snake is a serpent which goes along with its head up and its breast advanced. It is rarely seen but you can tell where it has passed along. These snakes are not thought to be very long, but they appear to vary in size. The largest would probably measure a foot and a half in diameter. With its sharp breast this snake tears up the earth, making a deep furrow. It is supposed to be covered with a crust of scales, and where it has touched against stones, and even rocks, it can be seen that they give way to its great power. It can cut through the roots of trees, making the trees keel over, and throw mud high up on the trunks of trees near by. These snakes, when they move in this way, appear to be changing their places of residence and this is always done during a rainstorm. You can see where lightning has struck all along where this snake has been. Such things prove to the Indians that such a snake exists. A Choctaw Indian named John Wesley, in the old Choctaw country south of the Canadian, told Lewis that one of these snakes had in some way been mortally wounded and lay up in the mountains. A number of people saw it and told Wesley about it, and he thought of going to see it but did not. The snake lay there until it was dead, however, and the skeleton was seen by people and spoken of frequently. Wesley knew where this could be found and told Lewis that if he came over they would go over there together and see the bones, but Lewis did not go. This happened in 1905.

---

47 For another version see pp. 71–72.   48 Ms., Bur. Amer. Ethn.

The origin of the conception of this snake is without doubt to be found in the tracks made by lightning, and the bones supposed to have been left by one of them might well have been those of some animal exposed at the time of a thundershower.

The horned snake was probably held in highest esteem by the Indians on account of the value placed upon its horns as hunting charms. The following account of it is mainly from Jackson Lewis. This snake lives in water and has horns like the stag. It is not a bad snake. It crawls out and suns itself near its hole, and on one occasion Lewis claimed to have seen such a snake. It does not harm human beings but seems to have a magnetic power over game. If any game animal, such as a deer, comes near the place where this snake is lying it is drawn irresistibly into the water and destroyed. It eats only the ends of the noses of the animals which it has killed. The old Creeks sometimes got hold of the horns of this snake, and they were broken up into very minute fragments and distributed among the hunters of the Creek Nation. These fragments are red and look like red sealing wax. A Creek hunter is always exceedingly anxious to obtain even the most minute fragment of such a horn, because it is said to give luck and success in hunting and killing deer. "I myself," said Lewis, "have at two times in my life owned a small fragment of one of these horns, and as you yourself know [speaking to Mr. G. W. Grayson] I have always been looked upon as a great deer killer." These snakes are very rarely seen.

The Alabama living in Texas also know of this snake, which they call tcinto sáktco, "crawfish (i. e. long-horned) snake." They say they are of four kinds according as their horns are yellow, white, red, or blue.

Tuggle makes mention of another snake described as living under ground. "It is never seen, but it emerges sometimes from the ground, with a great noise, and leaves a large hole in the earth where it came out. It is called the Celestial One, or Good Snake." [49] This snake is probably identical with that described by Jackson Lewis, a most remarkable snake, since it consists principally of head and lacks a body. It lives on the dew from the grass and leaves. It swirls round and round in the air and goes upward until it disappears, from which fact it would seem to typify the whirlwind.

Jackson Lewis told me of a certain set of supernatural beings residing in the waters and therefore called "the inhabitants of the waters." One of these was the horned snake already mentioned. A second was "the long snake," which coils itself up round and round to a height of perhaps 3 feet. This is perhaps identical with the snake which produces thunder. Another was "the great yellow snake," which is under the ground ordinarily but also burrows its way into

---

[49] Tuggle, Ms., Bur. Amer. Ethn.

the waters. Still another was a snake as large around as a stovepipe. Several of these sometimes get together and raise themselves straight up until they can not go higher, when they fall over with a splash. Occasionally they sport in the water by extending themselves across running water in the form of a bow and bending back and forth while the water roars over them. According to Lewis these snakes seem to be chiefs among all the inhabitants of the waters. Other "inhabitants of the waters" are the water bear, water calf, water bison, water tiger, and water person. The water tiger is spotted like a leopard, and is now often identified with that animal.[50] The water person is about 4 feet tall and has long hair.

My Natchez informant had heard a tradition that his people once worshiped a snake to which the women gave their children as food from time to time, but this seems to be a modern myth about the doings of the remote ancestors which has secured a foothold among several tribes.

There are many stories about a monster lizard supposed to live like a bear in hollow trees. It is called by the same name, atcukliba, as a small, inoffensive striped lizard found on trees. It is related that at one time some hunters were encamped near the tree in which such a giant lizard lived. One of the men "had a word," that is a formula of supernatural power, and he said that he could get the best of this animal. He went to the place where it lived and shouted "Come out. We will race." Immediately the atcukliba came out and started in pursuit of the man who ran on across country uttering a peculiar yell. The lizard was close behind him, but the man kept ahead until they were out of sight. By and by the people saw them coming back, the man still in the lead, and, when they got near, the lizard was so much exhausted that it had to lie down. Later a man without power thought he could do the same thing. He kept ahead of the lizard until they were out of sight, but when it was time for them to reappear they saw the atcukliba coming with the man in its mouth. Upon this the onlookers set the woods on fire so that the creature could not pursue them and fled. This lizard appears also in the tales of the Texas Alabama.

The eagle and a small sparrow hawk that eats chickens each receives the name of "the king of birds." The feathers of the former were highly prized, and were used in dances and games, particularly by members of the Tciloki clans; from this and other circumstances it is evident that it was a war emblem. Adair says that the whole town would contribute, "to the value of 200 deer-skins," to the killing of a large eagle, and the man who did so received an honorable title for the exploit, just as if he had brought in the scalp of an enemy. The bald-headed eagle was not esteemed. According

---

[50] A famous story in which this snake figures has been given on pp. 70, 71 of the preceding paper.

to Adair all of the Indian nations with which he was familiar considered the raven impure, yet had a kind of superstitious regard for it.[51] Crow feathers were among the war feathers of the Creeks.

Among the Texas Alabama the hoot owl (o'pa) informed prophets when a death or some other misfortune was about to take place. A man who was fond of joking and a prophet were once out hunting when one of these birds flew near and hooted. The former then asked the prophet in a jesting way if he knew what the owl said, and the prophet answered, "He said another man is going with your wife." Upon this the jester cut 12 long sticks, went home, found that the prophet had spoken truly, and beat the guilty pair in accordance with native custom. My informant seemed to think that in cases of death the owl was the man's soul, but this is doubtful. Another prophetic bird was a small red-headed woodpecker having speckled wings which makes a noise resembling bicici, and is hence called in Alabama bicici'hka. When the nephew of one of my informants died, the wife of the former was away in a river bottom. While she was there and before the news had reached her she saw one of these birds flying about. Adair tells us that on one occasion he observed the Indians "to be intimidated at the voice of a small uncommon bird, when it perched, and chirped on a tree over their war camp." [52] This may have been one of the birds above mentioned or a third of similar character.

Dogs are sometimes fabled to have helped men and there are stories which represent them as living in towns with square grounds like those of human beings. It is said that upon one occasion a boy found a deserted house in which was a bitch with a litter of puppies. He took care of them, and when the pups grew up they went out and drove bear up to him so that he could shoot them with arrows. The skunk is once referred to as "chief of all the animals." [52a]

As stated in the beginning, supernatural power of some sort was believed to attach to all animals and plants, and to natural objects generally, even to artificial objects, and when we come to discuss Creek medicine a great deal more will be said about their various powers, because each is supposed to have been able to produce certain diseases.

Some mythic supernatural beings have already been mentioned, but there were a number of others, many of which caused sickness. Among these were a race of little people, called by Tuggle "fairies." [53] They lived in hollow trees, on tree tops, in the holes in the rocks, and in other similar places. They were strong and handsome, with fine figures, and sometimes they allowed themselves to be seen by a human being, who then talked about them continually

---

[51] Adair, Hist. Am. Inds., pp. 131, 173, 194.
[52] Ibid., p. 26.
[52a] See p. 529.
[53] Tuggle, Ms., Bur. Amer. Ethn.

and followed wherever they led, into forests, swamps, etc. Sometimes the victim died in these desolate spots, but at others he came to his senses and got back home. The mental disease which they thus induced seems to have been a kind of temporary insanity. They rather bewildered the victim, then put him permanently out of his head. One man told me he had been led astray twice by these beings; they conducted him across a river in this state, and he was never able to explain how he got there. This was a favorite trick of the little people.

Once, when the father of one of my Natchez informants was out hunting, and could get nothing, he heard little people calling to him. He could not see them until he looked down near the ground. They wore caps and some had bows and arrows. They directed him to a place where medicine was to be found and to a place where there was game, so he followed their directions. First he found a little stone cup filled with medicine which he drank, and then he went on and killed a deer.

There were also giants whose eyes opened vertically instead of horizontally. They treated human beings in the same way as the little people. The Choctaw and Chickasaw have the same beliefs regarding giants and dwarfs as have the Creeks.

There is supposed to be an animal called hàtcko-tcápko—"long ears." It is about the size of a mule, has immense ears, and a very hideous appearance generally. It has a disagreeable odor and causes a dangerous disease, but fortunately it is rarely seen. There are two varieties of this animal, one of a brown color nearly black, the other of a slate color.

Another creature is called nokos oma, "like a bear." It is of about the size of an ordinary black bear, but it always carries its head near the earth. It has immense tusks which cross each other and when seen it is going along a trail with the gait of a pacer. More often, however, only the noise made by the males is heard, and this sounds something like "kàp kàp kàp kàp."

The hàtcko fàski, "sharp ears," seem to go in pairs and never travel east or west but always north or south. They are observed especially near the sources of small streams. They have sharp noses, bushy tails, and globular feet.

There are some animals, usually pied in color, which look like big steers. They are called wak oma, "like a cow." Several travel together and they move in single file and alternately. One moves on for a certain distance and stops and then moves on again. The one behind moves up to the place which the first had occupied, stops, and moves on again in the same manner.

There is an animal called lohka which sometimes appears in the shape of a cat, sometimes as a chicken.

There is also a bird called so'datcă'kală which never looks toward the earth but always straight up into the sky. It makes a noise like a woodpecker, and my informant thought he had heard it at times in the dead hours of the night far up in the air.

Another bird is like a woodpecker but much larger. It lives in pine forests, but the old doctors when they made medicine, and had occasion to refer to it, sang of it as if it originated in the skies. These two last may be real creatures, the former the "sun gazer," the latter a woodpecker.

There was said to be a little deer about 2 feet high and either speckled like a fawn or white, but it differed from a fawn in having very lofty horns. This is called "the chief deer." My informant claimed to have killed one of these.

The water king deer (Wiofû'tc miko) is mentioned as causing certain diseases, and Speck's informant attributed others to the "sky-hog" and the "wolf-in-the-water."

There is also mention of the "spirit of war," which appears to have been in human shape.

Besides the above, in the doctoring formulæ and in the myths we hear of a cat-like creature called isti-papa, "man-eater." This is usually identified with the "lion," while the panther is commonly referred to as a "tiger." It is possible that the conception may have come in after white contact, but on the other hand it might preserve a memory of the jaguar which anciently came as far north as the Brazos River and probably to the Mississippi. The Alabama identify the "man-eater" (Ala. atipa-tcoba) with the elephant, of which they had of course no knowledge until late times.

Alabama Indians also told of certain beings with penises so long that they reached high up into the trees; they were in the habit of striking the trees with these and the noise resulting could be heard for long distances.

The monsters of Muskhogean legend frequently trail their intended victims by means of a roller which is spoken of as if it were endowed with a conscious or semiconscious life of its own. It is described in one place as about 3 inches in diameter and the idea of it is evidently derived from the roller formerly used in the chunkey game.[53a]

CHARMS

Among these objects, which are rather means of securing supernatural help than active helpers themselves, the sabīa were the most important, and they are said to be known to all of the Five Civilized Tribes. I have heard of them personally among the Creeks, Alabama, and Natchez. They were very small objects looking like crystals and when properly treated would bring the possessor success in any

---

[53a] See p. 466 in the preceding paper.

emergency of life, in public speaking and in war, but particularly in hunting and in love. If the owner of a sabīa asked for a thing he would never be refused. The Texas Alabama claim that with them it was only a love charm and had nothing to do with hunting. However, it was a saying that anything that will charm a deer will charm a woman. The word is said to convey the impression of a group of men starting off carrying some particular article, but its origin may have had nothing to do with this. The best account of it was obtained from Jackson Lewis, and in substance it is as follows:

There are different kinds of sabīa—white, blue, red, yellow, and one that is nearly black. All have a luster like that of glass except the black, which looks like the graphite of a lead pencil. The red and yellow sabīa are considered the strong ones or the males; the white and blue are the females. If one sits down and watches them a moment they gleam and flash as if they were live things moving about. Lewis owned a white sabīa and also a blue one for a long time but sold them when he partially lost his eyesight. Upon one occasion he took one of these out, laid it upon the table, and was about to touch it with the point of his penknife when it sprang off to a distance of 2 or 3 feet like a thing alive. According to tradition sabīa and the knowledge of how they should be used came from the Yamasee, so that in singing the long song which goes with them, but is not used much on account of its sacredness, the word Yamasee continually occurs. The sabīa was kept in a little piece of buckskin along with red paint, and when a man went out hunting he opened this up, took a little red paint out on the end of a match or straw, and put it on his cheek. Then the deer did not seem wild and there was little trouble experienced in finding and shooting them. This is not done until one has gotten a little distance from camp, and the action is accompanied by a song intended to make the deer approach. Another song may be sung to blind the deer after one has seen him so that you can get as near to him as possible before shooting. During the sabīa songs the charm itself is not unwrapped. Some sabīa now in use are said to have been obtained from the Yamasee, while others are reputed to have been borne upon a plant which grows in out-of-the-way places. This plant has minute seeds which fall off when they are ripe and form such crystals. Numerous songs were connected with this charm, and it is said that "one could never finish telling the myths concerning it." Sometimes a sabīa is found whirling around on gravelly or sandy soil and acting as if it were alive

Another man, who claimed merely to have seen imitations of the yellow and blue varieties but not the true sabīa, said that they were so powerful that the owner would not keep one in the house. It was put in the middle of a circular piece of buckskin taken from the flank of a deer and tied up tight until it was to be used. When a hunter having one of these failed to kill a deer and the sun was already high in the heavens he untied this charm and held it in his hand so that the rays of the sun might fall upon it. Then he sang a song to it which made it wriggle in the paint. Forthwith the deer would be charmed and would sometimes come straight toward the hunter. This man, it is to be noted, differs from Jackson Lewis regarding the unwrapping of the sabía. He was less likely to be correct, but on the other hand there were probably many different ways of treatment.

Cook said that unless it is carefully handled and controlled by the right formula the sabía will injure its owner by exciting him "sexually" or affecting his wife and daughters in the same manner. Therefore it was generally not carried on the person unless its owner was ready for an emergency and had his formula constantly in mind, which makes it entirely safe. It is easily lost, and will jump away quickly. The roots of the sabía hálgi ("sabía wife") were also used as a charm. This is one of the first plants to come out in spring. These charms are still in use, being employed largely as love charms.

Still another informant suggested that the "fox fire" sometimes seen in punk perhaps originated the sabía idea; the phosphorescent light was associated with the daylight luster of these crystals and hence supposed to be self-derived—i. e., the result of a volitional act on the part of the stone. The following account of the plant and mineral sabías is from the Tuggle collection:

"A man once went to the woods and remained in solitary meditation for four days. He wandered alone till he heard a soft, low, sweet voice, singing a song. He listened and watched. He saw a beautiful little flower, swaying gracefully back and forth. He knew the song came from the little flower. Around the flower the ground was swept clean. He listened until he had learned the song. Suddenly he felt that he possessed a wonderful power, which he could impart to any object. Any one who had such an object in his possession became lucky. He could succeed in love, in the chase, and in war. Often bits of stone possess this power. The color of these charmed stones is white, red, and yellow. They are called 'Sar-pee-yah.'" [54]

One of the vegetable sabías was called sabía hagi ("like a sabía"). It has a globular root and a white flower, said to be the first flower to appear in spring. When a man discovered such a plant he set up a stake near by to mark it so that he could dig it up when it got big enough. That time having arrived, the prospective owner went to the river and dived into it four times. Then he procured a piece of white buckskin, put some red paint on this, and placed the root on the paint. It was then laid away carefully in a secure, dry place

---

[54] Tuggle, Ms , Bur. Amer. Ethn.

away from the house, for if it were in the latter place the whole family would go wild and act like deer at the rutting season. When the owner wanted to go hunting he took a little paint from around the root and put it on his face, and if he were going far the whole charm could be carried along.

Another sabīa was known as sabīa hàtki ("white sabīa"). It has small leaves and a bunch of black berries at the top, and grows to the height of about 1½ feet. If a man chewed a little of this when he was out hunting he would immediately encounter a deer. It also had power to attract women.

The sabīa crystal was, at least by some, believed to come from a plant. This is shown by the following account of this charm taken down by Mr. G. W. Grayson from an Indian doctor, Caley Proctor, the use of which has been kindly allowed me by Mr. Grayson's family.

"The subbea is often found in the bulb of a rare plant. The plant is never found growing abundantly in any locality. It is pulled from the ground and from the bulb is stripped off each outer coating until the center is reached when there will be found something, a very small piece of broken glass, red, amber, or of some other color. It is taken out and put into a small quantity of red paint, and the whole is securely wrapped in a small piece of white dressed buckskin. This is the famous subbea, especially useful in giving luck to hunters who know the song and sing it to the enclosed subbea, or success to him who desires to win the affections of one of the opposite sex."

Jackson Lewis had heard of two other roots used by the Creeks in hunting, though they were not spoken of as sabīas. One he had never seen. The other was a very small plant with a very small bulbous root. The root is rubbed over the eyelashes two ways, horizontally and vertically, when it produces success in hunting. If one has had bad or inauspicious dreams during the night and does not feel encouraged to go out hunting these bulbs will free him of this feeling and "set him up" for the day.

A third root had been obtained from the wild tribes of the west. If one made lines with this one on the face and hands and a straight mark on the bottom of the foot he would have good luck. It would also stop nosebleed. The western Indians claim that when they administer it to a horse about to run a race the horse always wins. Jackson Lewis himself once had a piece of this medicine and testified to its power.

As a charm against snake bite they hung the thigh bone of the highland terrapin about the necks of children.

Adair speaks of a beaded string of bison hair which Indian women tied around their legs as "a great ornament, as well as a preservative against miscarriages, hard labor, and other evils."[55]

---

55 Adair, Hist. Am. Inds., p. 169.

When a nail or some similar object was run into the body the red-headed woodpecker called tītka was used as a charm to get it out.

The "ark" which they carried to war was another kind of charm. When they defeated the French under D'Artaguette they insisted on killing the priests because they believed the articles for the performance of the mass which the latter carried were the French ark and the priests its keepers.[56]

A piece of the horn of a horned snake was one of the greatest charms. Some men claimed that they had been able to charm such a snake by their songs so as to bring it to the bank of the stream, when they obtained a piece of one of its horns. This was kept in a hollow tree or some other place remote from the house lest it should make the children sick.[56a]

An Alabama hunter carried a piece of the root of the wàtola im-bàkca ("crane's cord") in his ball pouch, and if he could not find deer he would sing and talk to it, blow upon it, and then chew it. Then he was sure to find and kill the animals.

Bartram speaks of the "physic-nut, or Indian olive" as similarly used, and says: "The Indians when they go in pursuit of deer carry this fruit with them, supposing that it has the power of charming or drawing that creature to them.[57] Although the identification is a little uncertain this seems to be the fruit of the *Triosteum perfoliatum* or "horse gentian."

The early white traders were often so affected by native superstitions regarding charms that they placed unbounded confidence in them themselves. Thus Adair says that he took the foot of a "guinea deer" out of the shot pouch of one of these men "and another from my own partner, which they had very safely sewed in the corner of each of their otter-skin pouches, to enable them, according to the Indian creed, to kill deer, bear, buffalo, beaver, and other wild beasts in plenty." Argument proving unavailing he was constrained to return them to their owners lest an accident might befall them and the blame be laid upon him.[58]

At times, it would seem, an Indian would turn upon his charm and throw it away if it did not appear to him to be sufficiently active in his behalf. Adair mentions a case in which an Upper Creek Indian burned himself so badly in the fire when under the influence of liquor that he became furiously angry with it, upbraiding it for its treatment of him after all of the food he had given it. It is added that from then on he became godless, though perhaps only with respect to that particular element. Adair says that he had witnessed several instances of "impiety" of like nature.[59]

[56] Adair, Hist. Am. Inds., pp. 154–155. See pp. 411–412, 425.
[56a] See p. 429.
[57] Bartram, Travels, p. 41.
[58] Adair, op. cit., p. 239.
[59] Ibid., p. 116. Also see p. 484.

Magical songs or formulas accompanied the use of most medicines and charms, and very wonderful things were supposed to be accomplished by these. "By a word" a man could stand aside in the warpath and render himself invisible to the enemies. "By a word" a man could even condense the whole world in such a way that he could go around it in four steps. A certain Indian in recent times "conjured" his field and sprinkled it with miko hoyanĭdja, and, "while the crops all about were ruined, he had a good harvest."

Tribal medicines or palladia such as are often met with in other parts of America were almost unknown to the Creeks unless we include the "ark" or war medicine under this head. Adair and some later writers mention a human figure carved out of wood in one of the upper towns,[60] and I myself was told of a wooden eagle with drops of blood represented issuing from the corners of its mouth which was brought out and planted in front of the miko's bed at Coweta when anything of importance was to be discussed. The Creek chief James Islands spoke of articles used by various towns during the celebration of the busk and held in great reverence, and he instanced large conch shells out of which the Coweta Indians took their black drink. These, he said, they had had for a long time and preserved with great care. But there is no certainty that these things were really palladia. Nevertheless, there is one apparent exception, the famous copper and brass plates preserved by the town of Tukabahchee. Hitchcock says that, in his time, these were kept in a small house which stood by itself tightly shut up, situated near the tcokofa, but at a later period, and apparently at an earlier one also, they were in the sanctuary behind the middle section of the Chiefs' bed. The small detached houses, such as Hitchcock describes, were built in several of the square grounds and I have seen some of them, but I was given to understand that they represented a recent institution, being used probably as a protection against the all-consuming curiosity of the white man. The plates were brought out once annually at the time of the busk and formed the principal feature in one of their dances to be described presently. The first account of them that has come down to us is by, or rather through, Adair and is of the utmost importance. It runs as follows:

"In the Tuccabatches on the Tallapoose river, thirty miles above the Allabahamah garrison, are two brazen tablets, and five of copper. They esteem them so sacred as to keep them constantly in their holy of holies, without touching them in the least, only in the time of their compounded first-fruit-offerings, and annual expiation of sins; at which season, their magus carries one under his arm, a-head of the people, dancing round the sacred arbour; next to him their head-warrior carries another; and those warriors who chuse it,

---

[60] Adair, Hist. Am. Inds., pp. 22–23.

carry the rest after the manner of the high priest; all the others carry white canes with swan-feathers at the top. Hearing accidentally of these important monuments of antiquity, and enquiring pretty much about them, I was certified of the truth of the report by four of the southern traders, at the most eminent Indian trading house of all English America. One of the gentlemen informed me, that at my request he endeavoured to get a liberty of viewing the aforesaid tables, but it could not possibly be obtained, only in the time of the yearly grand sacrifice, for fear of polluting their holy things, at which time gentlemen of curiosity may see them. *Old Bracket*, an Indian of perhaps 100 years old, lives in that old beloved town, who gave the following description of them:

"*Old Bracket's* account of the *five copper* and *two brass* plates under the beloved cabbin in Tuccabatchey-square.

 The shape of the five copper plates; one is a foot and a half long and seven inches wide, the other four are shorter and narrower.

The largest stamped thus: Æ   The shape of the two brass plates,—about a foot and a half in diameter.

"He said he was told by his forefathers that those plates were given to them by the man we call God; that there had been more of other shapes, some as long as he could stretch with both his arms, and some had writing upon them which were buried with particular men; and that they had instructions given with them, viz. they must only be handled by particular people, and those fasting; and no unclean woman must be suffered to come near them or the place where they are deposited. He said, none but this town's people had any such plates given them, and that they were a different people from the Creeks. He only remembered three more, which were buried with three of his family, and he was the only man of the family now left. He said, there were two copper plates under the king's cabin, which had lain there from the first settling of the town.

"This account was taken in the Tuccabatchey-square, 27th July, 1759, per Will. Bolsover." [61]

Swan, writing in 1791, mentions them again in these words:

"There are preserved in the Tuckabatches' town, on the Tallapoosee river, some thin pieces of wrought brass, found in the earth when the Indians first dug for clay to build in this place. Nobody can tell how long since they were dug up; but the Indians preserve them as proofs of their right to the ground, having descended to them by their departed ancestors, from time immemorial." [62]

---

[61] Note in Adair, pp. 178–179.   [62] Swan in Schoolcraft, Ind. Tribes, vol. v, p. 283.

If Swan means that the plates had been dug up at the place where the Tukabahchee then were he is in error, since the tribe had occupied that place probably not a hundred years. He may have been led into a misunderstanding owing to the fact that some of them were buried in the earth, under the Chiefs' bed.[63] Pickett gives the following account of the ceremony observed in carrying them beyond the Mississippi at the time of the Creek removal:

"When the inhabitants of this town, in the autumn of 1836, took up the line of march for their present home in the Arkansas Territory, these plates were transported thence by six Indians, remarkable for their sobriety and moral character, at the head of whom was the Chief, Spoke-oak, Micco [Ispokōgi miko].[64] Medicine, made expressly for their safe transportation, was carried along by these warriors. Each one had a plate strapped behind his back, enveloped nicely in buckskin. They carried nothing else, but marched on, one before the other, the whole distance to Arkansas, neither communicating nor conversing with a soul but themselves, although several thousands were emigrating in company; and walking, with a solemn religious air, one mile in advance of the others."[65] As to their origin he says:

"Another tradition is, that the Shawnees gave these plates to the Tookabatchas, as tokens of their friendship, with an injunction that they would annually introduce them in their religious observances of the new corn season. But the opinion of Opothleoholo, one of the most gifted of the modern Creeks, went to corroborate the general tradition that they were gifts from the Great Spirit."[65]

Most of this information was obtained from Barent Dubois, whom Pickett describes as "an intelligent New Englander"[66] but Schoolcraft terms a citizen of New York.[67] There is no doubt of its substantial accuracy. What he says regarding the manner of transporting the plates west is confirmed by General Hitchcock on the authority of a half-breed Creek chief who told him that "when the general emigration took place in 1836 a number of people were selected to convey those articles to the west and they went in advance of the nation. No man was allowed to precede the party in charge of those articles."[67a]

Schoolcraft includes a particular account of the plates in the third volume of his great work, and adds a little information which we may infer from the context was obtained from Walter Lowrie, Esq., president of the Presbyterian Board of Foreign Missions, who

---

[63] See p. 504.
[64] This was not the town chief but a chief who seems to have had peculiar priestly functions. See p. 66.
[65] Pickett, Hist. Ala., vol. I, pp. 86–87. Charleston, 1851.
[66] Ibid., p. 87.
[67] Schoolcraft, Ind. Tribes, vol. III, p. 90.
[67a] Hitchcock, Ms. notes.

examined them in the Choctaw country in 1852. According to this statement "Muscogee tradition affirms that there were more of these plates possessed by them at former periods, of different kinds, some of which had letters or figures, but that the number was diminished by the custom of placing one or more of them with the body of a deceased chief of the pure or reigning blood. The plates remaining are placed in the hands of particular men. They are guarded with care, and kept from being touched by women." He repeats the tradition that they had been derived from the Shawnee, which I also heard. It was supposed that they were handed down from above and given to the Shawnee who turned them over to the Ispokogi. Schoolcraft's reproductions of these plates agree substantially with those of Adair, except that the letters are placed nearer the center of the "shield," and the two black dots are shown clearly to have been intended for holes. They were based on information furnished by the Walter Lowrie above mentioned.[68]

A second account appears in the Appendix to the fifth volume of Schoolcraft contributed by the Creek missionary Loughridge, joint author of a dictionary of the Creek language. It is as follows:

TULLAHASSEE MISSION,
Creek Agency, W. Ark., 14th Sept., 1852.[69]

Having understood that the Tukkabachee town or clan of Creek Indians, were holding their annual festival, ("the green corn dance,") and that they would exhibit the much talked of "brass plates," I determined to examine them, and therefore proceeded to their town, and camped for the night, on the 7th of August, 1850.

Before daylight next morning, I was aroused by the singing, dancing and whooping, of the Indians, and was informed that the dance with the plates had commenced.

"On reaching the place, I found 200 or 300 men assembled in the Square, with fires burning to give them light. About 80 or 100 of them were formed into a procession, marching with a dancing step, double file, around their "stamping ground," which is about 240 feet in circumference. The procession was led by seven men, each of whom carried one of the plates with much solemnity of manner. After the dance was over, (which lasted about an hour,) I sent in my request for permission to inspect the plates.

"The old chief Tukkabachee Mikko, came out and said that I could see them, on condition that *I would not touch them.* They profess to believe, that if any person who has not been consecrated for the purpose, by fasting or other exercises, six or eight days, should touch them, he would certainly die, and sickness or some great calamity would befall the town. For similar reasons, he said it was unlawful

---

[68] Schoolcraft, Ind. Tribes, vol. III, pp 87-90.   [69] Ibid., vol. v, p. 660.

for a woman to look at them. The old chief then conducted me into the square, or public ground, where the plates had been laid out for my inspection. There were seven in all, three brass and four copper plates.

"The brass plates are circular, very thin, and are, respectively about twelve, fourteen, and eighteen inches in diameter. The middle sized one has two letters (or rather a double letter) near its centre, about one-fourth of an inch in length; thus, Æ, very well executed, as if done by a stamp. This was the only appearance of writing which I could discern on any of them.

"The four copper plates (or strips) are from four to six inches in width, and from one and a half to two feet in length. There is nothing remarkable about them. Like the brass plates, they are very thin, and appear as if they had been cut out of some copper kettle or other vessel.

"The Indians cannot give any satisfactory account of any of these plates. They say that they have been handed down from father to son, for many generations past, as relics of great value, on account of the blessing supposed to be attached to the proper attention to them. They hold, that the health and prosperity of the town, depend in a great measure upon the proper observance of the rites connected with them. It is said, that this town is known to have had these plates in their possession for 200 years past.

"There has been much conjecture about the writing upon them. Some supposed that it was Hebrew, and hence concluded that they might be descendants of the Jews. I was, therefore, the more anxious to see the plates, and very particular in examining them. But I could discover no appearance of writing, and not a single letter, but the above mentioned Roman letters.

"Some have supposed the brass plates to be old shields. The largest one, (which I could not examine very closely), appeared more like the remains of a shield than any of them.

"But upon the whole, I am inclined to adopt the opinion given me by one of their dancers in the procession, that *"they appear to have been covers for pots, or for some other vessel, taken a great while ago from the Spaniards perhaps, in Florida."*

"Yours truly,

R. M. LOUGHRIDGE."

Stiggins's account of them again brings in the Shawnee:

"It is related that once in times past, the Ispocoga and Shawanose tribes, made a resolution and formed a compact by which they were thereafter to consolidate their interests and the two tribes to be but one in future, and perform their yearly custom of Thanksgiving and other rites of religious ceremony as one people. For they at that [time] lived bordering on each other's Territory, the Shawanose in and about Savannah in the state of Georgia, therefore, in accordance with their compact, they deposited with the keepers of the national square of one of the tribes, their calumet tobacco pipes, belts, and war club called by them *Attussa*, with all their emblems of peace and friendship together with twelve pieces of brass described as follows: Six of them were oval of about eight inches long and seven in the widest part and the other six about nine inches long and four in width, made square, bearing a resemblance to the breast plates of ancient soldiers. They all belonged to the Ispocoga tribe, and were three of the oval and three of the square kind making six to a set when exhibited for they are never exhibited but in their fasting and feasting to commemorate the new corn crop. So they deposited two sets of the above plates in the national square according to compact, and the united tribes of Ispocoga and Shawanose performed their ceremonies together with concord for a length of time. But for some unknown reason or on account of some occurrence—the Ispocogas attributing it to the instable and fickle disposition of the Shawanose—the latter formed a resolution to secede from the union and national compact and remove. No remonstrance of the other tribe against it could alter their determination for they dissolved their union by emigrating northwardly, and when they moved they carried off six of the sacred brass plates, three oval and three of the square kinds, which the Shawanose have retained possession of ever since. They were seen by some Creeks first in the care of the old prophet at Tippacanoe about the time he fought Genl. Harrison and not long since they were still in his possession over the Mississippi, and seen by some Creek chiefs who visited that tribe, to whom they were exhibited with a traditional account of how they came into their possession with all its circumstances, which account agreed with the Ispocoga tradition of their loss." [70]

Although there are other incidental references to these plates, including several newspaper accounts of more or less value, the only one with which we need concern ourselves is that given by Tuggle and preserved among the ethnological papers in the Bureau of American Ethnology. I quote it entire:

"The Tookabatchees have in their possession certain copper or brass vessels, which their town has owned for generations . . .

"These sacred vessels consist of twelve pieces. The largest is circular in shape, about eighteen inches in diameter and has two holes near the center through which a string passes. Two other pieces are circular and about fifteen inches in diameter with two holes near the center. Nine other pieces are smaller, being twelve or fifteen inches long and six inches wide.

"The Tookabatchees give the following account of the origin of these vessels:

---

[70] Stiggins, Ms.

" 'A long time ago Is-poke-o-goes, persons, came from Esar-kee-tum-mee-see, the Life Controller, Source of Life, and brought the vessels to us. After staying some time one of the "Is-poke-o-gees" went back to Esarkee-tum-meesee. The other Ispokegee remained with our people. He was without beginning. He told us always to preserve these vessels and carry them wherever we went. He told us how to live and do right and tell the truth. He told us that after a while a great many white people would come from the east and drive us away, but always to carry these vessels and good luck would be with us, in hunting and in war. He told us that the Shawnees also had such vessels and some day they would unite with us and we would be one people.

" 'The Ispokeogee took the wrong medicine and died. Four days after he was buried, a beautiful white flower was seen growing on his grave and from this flower the Tookabatchees obtained their medicine (the wild tobacco), and keep it to this day.

" 'These vessels are kept buried under the town house and at the busk, or annual festival, they are unearthed, washed in a running stream, and rubbed by certain persons to whom they are entrusted, and they are used during the festival for certain ceremonies. When the festival is over the seed of their medicine is put with these sacred vessels, and they are returned to their hiding till the next annual busk.'

"Strangers can not look on these vessels except at the festival and it is claimed that should a stranger look on them at other times he would die before he reached his home."

In some notes made by Mr. G. W. Grayson after a visit to the Tukabahchee busk of 1917 occurs the following reference to these plates:

"The Indians declare they were given to them from on high at a very early period of their existence as a people, and attribute to them profound sacredness. From such information as I have been able to secure respecting these curious objects it would seem that some 70 or more years ago they were much more come-at-able, in other words that the custodians were more readily induced to permit them to be seen than in later times. I find that the present custodians appear to regard them with a degree of awe that is more pronounced than in earlier periods. It is asserted that these objects have not been disturbed or removed from their present inclosure for many years because, as it was explained, the old medicine men who by their powers of magic could handle them without detrimental consequences had all passed away. It seems to be firmly believed that should they now be taken out or handled by persons untaught in the mysteries and magic of the old medicine men of the past, dire results such as sickness in inordinate degrees of virulence, fatalities in the families of the town, destructive wind storms, and various other sinister phenomena would occur. So, when one was asked why they did not take the plates out and wash and brighten them up as was the early practice, the answer came promptly, 'Because there is none competent.' They must neither be handled nor touched by water lest great evils result. Moreover, they seem to speak of them with care and caution, closely bordering on fear, lest some evil befall them as a punishment for having spoken too freely of such sacred objects."

But some of these plates are now reported to be broken and parts lost, which is not to be wondered at, as for a long time they were kept in a box back of the miko's bed, along with the atasa carried by the women, exposed to any inquisitive passer-by not overblessed with scruples. In 1914, however, they were still held in the greatest esteem and fear by the leading Tukabahchee. The chief of the town at that time said he could never handle them without becoming sick, and when I drew outlines of the plates from my memory of Adair's figures he recommended that I tear them up and throw them away or ill would certainly befall me before I got home. The continued handling is supposed to drive one crazy. If some of these are brass, as stated by Adair and conceded by subsequent writers who have had a chance to examine the plates, the European origin of at least a portion of them is assured, and it is plainly indicated also by the letters, if they have been correctly copied. Barent Dubois, mentioned above in the quotation from Pickett, who is said by him to have "long lived among the Tookabatchas," believed that these plates owed their origin to De Soto and his companions.[71] There can be little reasonable doubt that they are of Spanish origin, but, as the Shawnee and "Kaskinampos" [72] were trading at St. Augustine in the latter part of the seventeenth century it is equally possible that they were obtained there at that period. They share with certain objects among the Plains tribes in a veneration bestowed upon European articles when they first made their appearance, and which they would certainly have failed to elicit at a later time after that familiarity had developed that "breeds contempt."

THE FATE OF SOULS

According to Adair the good spirits of the world above attend and favor the virtuous while the bad spirits in the west accompany and have power over the vicious,[73] but this probably gives a somewhat distorted view of the actual native belief. It is probable that the good spirits of which he speaks included most of those who became human helpers, whether in the sky or in other parts of the universe,

[71] Pickett, Hist. Ala., p. 84.   [72] See Bull. 73. Bur. Amer. Ethn., p. 214.   [73] Adair, Hist. Am. Inds., p. 36.

while the bad spirits were the ghosts of the dead, or at any rate spirits associated with the western world through which the soul first passed. This is suggested by what he states immediately afterwards. "On which account, when any of their relations die, they immediately fire off several guns, by one, two, and three at a time, for fear of being plagued with the last troublesome neighbors [i. e., the evil spirits of the west]: all the adjacent towns also on the occasion, whoop and halloo at night; for they reckon, this offensive noise sends off the ghosts to their proper fixed places, till they return at some certain time, to repossess their beloved tract of land, and enjoy their terrestrial paradise." [74] The good spirits could be attached to individuals somewhat like the personal manitous of the Algonkian tribes. This is also made evident in the case of the Chickasaw by Adair, who says: "Several warriors have told me, that their *Nana Ishto-hoollo*, 'concomitant holy spirits,' or angels, have forewarned them, as by intuition, of a dangerous ambuscade, which must have been attended with certain death, when they were alone, and seemingly out of danger; and by virtue of the impulse, they immediately darted off, and, with extreme difficulty, escaped the crafty, pursuing enemy." [75] At the present time it is not thought that spiritual experiences are enjoyed by any except those who take the higher courses of training already spoken of, most of whom are doctors. It may be that the persons who gave the above information to Adair belonged to that class, or it may be that personal manitous were more widely enjoyed in primitive times than later became usual, but of this last there is no proof. Even in the cases of the graduates the power acquired through their training no longer appears to be associated with supernatural guardian spirits. Such, however, was evidently the case in former days.

The fear of ghosts expressed in the quotation from Adair given above was marked and has persisted down to our own times. Certain diseases, to be considered presently, are attributed to dead bodies. Anciently, when an Indian passed a graveyard, in order to drive away the ghosts he would take a little ginseng (hilis hátki) into his mouth, chew it, and spit it out on each side alternately until he had spit four times each way. People would not eat cold food that had been kept overnight for fear the ghosts had partaken of it. Sometimes encounters with ghosts were fatal. Thus there is a Texas-Alabama story about a man who went out to hunt raccoons and on the way was joined by a ghost under the guise of a person well known to him. By and by they saw a raccoon run up a tree, and the ghost climbed up and threw it down. Presently they came to a tree where there was another raccoon, and this time the man climbed up. After he had gotten up 30 feet or so the ghost shouted, "Look at me." The

⁷⁴ Adair, Hist. Am. Inds., p. 36.   ⁷⁵ Ibid,, p. 37.

man looked and discovered the nature of his companion.   Then he
began to climb down and when he was nearly to the ground took off
his moccasins and threw them, one in one direction and one in another.
The ghost, however, ran after the moccasins, picked them up, and
then pursued the man, whom he threw down and killed.

Speaking of the site of old Okmulgee, Adair says that the Indians
"strenuously aver, that when necessity forces them to encamp there,
they always hear, at the dawn of the morning, the usual noise of
Indians singing their joyful religious notes, and dancing, as if going
down to the river to purify themselves, and then returning to the
old town-house: with a great deal more to the same effect." [76]   Adair
adds that they attributed his own inability to hear such things to
the fact that he was "an obdurate infidel that way." [77]

Says Pope:

"The *Creeks* in approaching the Frontiers of *Georgia*, always encamp
on the right hand side of the Road or Path, assigning the left, as
ominous, to the *Larvæ* or Ghosts of their departed Heroes who have
either unfortunately lost their scalps, or remain unburied.   The
Ghost of an Hero in either Predicament, is refused Admittance into
the Mansions of Bliss, and sentenced to take up its invisible and
darksome Abode, in the dreary Caverns of the Wilderness; until the
Indignity shall be retaliated on the Enemy, by some of his surviving
Friends." [78]

Pope's authority is not the best, but this certainly establishes the
fact that the Creeks had the same belief as the Chickasaw regarding
the necessity of placating spirits of the slain.

Adair is probably correct in attributing fatalistic beliefs to the
southern Indians as to the time when each man's life was to come to
an end.   He says that they had a common proverb "*Neetak Intahāh*
[Ni'tak intaha], 'The days appointed, or allowed him, were finished'
[the days finished for him].   And this is their firm belief; for they
affirm, that there is a fixt time, and place, when, and where, every
one must die, without any possibility of averting it.   They frequently say, 'Such a one was weighed on the path, and made to be
light.'" [79]

He also says that many believed marriages to be equally fated. [80]

We learn from Adair, in places already quoted, that the Chickasaw
discharged guns and whooped in order to drive the ghost of a dead
man to his fixed abode, but that it was believed that if he had been
slain in war his soul would haunt the eaves of the house until equal
blood had been shed for him. [81]   All accounts agree that after the
soul had been induced to leave the neighborhood of his living relatives he traveled westward, passed under the sky and proceeded

---

[76] Adair, Hist. Am. Inds., p 36.   [78] Pope, Tour, pp. 63–64.   [80] Ibid., p. 26.
[77] Ibid., p 37.   [79] Adair, op. cit., p.33.   [81] Schoolcraft, Ind. Tribes, vol. I, p. 310.

upward upon it to the land of The One Above or the Breath Holder. The name "spirits' road" given to the milky way shows that this was regarded as the trail upon which they went.

The Alabama "land of the blest" was also above. Eakins says: "They say their paradise, or happy hunting-grounds, is above; but where, they have no definite idea."[82] Bossu obtained a longer if not a more accurate statement, without, however, any localization of the realms of the hereafter:

"I have asked them what they thought of the other world, and they have answered that if they have not taken away any other man's wife, if they have not committed theft, nor killed anyone during their lives, they will go after death into an extremely fertile country, where they will lack neither women nor good grounds for hunting, which will become very easy for them; that if on the other hand they have done foolish things, if they have made fun of the Great Spirit, they will go after death into a sterile country full of thorns and brambles, where there will be neither hunting nor women; this is all I have been able to learn concerning the belief of these people regarding the other life."[83]

According to the living Alabama, who perhaps preserve the ancient conception in the best form, the souls had to encounter several dangers on this journey. First they came to a body of water, but this divided to right and left at their approach. Next they reached a place where were great numbers of serpents. These they passed safely by wrapping bàksha branches about their bodies so that the fangs of the reptiles could not reach them. Finally they came to a place where a battle was in progress, but they avoided this by blowing out tobacco smoke which rendered them invisible. Still another danger to be encountered, in just what order with reference to the others I do not know, was a great eagle, and that this might be fought off a large "butcher knife" was buried with the body of the deceased. From the extent to which property was buried with the dead it is evident that this was also supposed to accompany them into the hereafter. According to my Alabama informants the ghost remains near its body for four days. Adair is our only early authority for the expected ultimate return of souls to earth,[84] but there appears to be no good reason to doubt that such an idea prevailed with certain Indians, and he is confirmed by the Chickasaw interviewed on Schoolcraft's behalf during the middle of last century. "They believe," he says, "that the spirits of all the Chickasaws will go back to Mississippi, and join the spirits of those that have died there; and then all the spirits will return to the west before the world is destroyed by fire."[85]

[82] Schoolcraft, Ind. Tribes, vol. I, p. 273.
[83] Bossu, Nouv. Voy., vol. II, pp. 48–49.
[34] Adair, Hist. Am. Inds., pp. 178, 182, 397.
[84] Schoolcraft, op. cit., vol. I, p. 310.

Bartram and Swan both testify to Creek belief in a future state of existence. The former says:

"They believe in a future state, where the spirit exists, which they call the world of spirits, where they enjoy different degrees of tranquility or comfort, agreeably to their life spent here: a person who in his life has been an industrious hunter, provided well for his family, an intrepid and active warrior, just, upright, and done all the good he could, will, they say, in the world of spirits, live in a warm, pleasant country, where are expansive, green, flowery savannas and high forests, watered with rivers of pure waters, replenished with deer, and every species of game; a serene, unclouded and peaceful sky; in short, where there is fulness of pleasure, uninterrupted." [86]

Says Swan:

"They believe there is a state of future existence, and that according to the tenor of their lives, they shall hereafter be rewarded with the privilege of hunting in the realm of the Master of Breath, or of becoming Seminoles in the regions of the old sorcerer.

"But as it is very difficult for them to draw any parallel between virtue and vice, they are most of them flattered with the expectation of hereafter becoming great war leaders, or swift hunters in the beloved country of the great Hesakkdum Esee." [87]

He adds elsewhere that the land of the good was "some distant, unknown region, where game is plenty, and goods are very cheap; where corn grows all the year round, and the springs of pure water are never dried up," while the other is "a great ways off, in some dismal swamp, which is full of galling briars," and that there is no game or bear's oil in all that country. [88]

In reply to the queries of Hawkins, Ifa hadjo, the great Medal chief of Tukabahchee, and speaker for the Creek Nation in the national council, affirmed that his people believed that "the spirit (po-yau-ficpchau [poya-fiktca]) goes the way the sun goes, to the west, and there joins its family and friends, who went before it." He also affirmed "that those who behaved well, are taken under the care of E-sau-ge-túh Emis-see and assisted; and that those who have behaved ill, are left there to shift for themselves; and that there is no other punishment." [89]

Upon the whole, it is rather likely that native belief postulated the alternative that some of the souls of the dead, necessarily the bad ones, would not get past the great eagle and the other dangers to be encountered on the way to the land of souls and would remain in the realm of ghosts and other evil spirits in the west, but the reward of the good hereafter was identified for the most part with

[86] Bartram, Travels, p. 496.
[87] Swan in Schoolcraft, Ind. Tribes, vol. V, p. 270.
[88] Ibid., pp. 269-270.
[89] Hawkins, Sketch, Ga. Hist. Soc. Colls., vol. III, p. 80.

their reward here, positions of esteem in the tribe, plenty to eat and wear, and plenty of enemies to kill, for the Creek social system rewarded so well in this world virtue of the kind these Indians recognized that it was not necessary to postpone all enjoyment of it to an uncertain hereafter.[90]

Bartram adds that according to native belief not merely man but every living creature had a spirit or soul that could exist apart from the body and that some had reported that "a pattern or spiritual likeness of everything living, as well as inanimate, exists in another world." [91] This, of course, is true of practically all primitive peoples, the only question being whether the term "other world" may be properly applied here.

MISCELLANEOUS BELIEFS

Dreams and visions seen in trances were one means of learning about the spirit world, and they were very generally credited. Bartram says: "They relate abundance of stories of men that have been dead or thought dead for many hours and days, who have revived again, giving an account of their transit to and from the world of souls, and describing the condition and situation of the place and spirits residing there." [91] A curious expression was used by the Creeks when they were about to go to bed. They would say Posálkan hoboyälänäs, "I am going to hunt a dream." If a man made a noise like an animal in his sleep those who heard him would say "that is his sleep (or dream) [inutcka, his sleep; imboitcka or imposálga, his dream]. If any person in a family dreamed of fire it foreboded sickness, especially bilious fever, and all of them took miko hoyanīdja and afterwards dipped in the creek four times. If they happened to have no medicine they at least bathed.

When a person sneezed it was supposed that someone was saying something good about him, and he would remark "Oh yes, that is what they always say about me." There is a jesting relation regarding a man who began sneezing and kept repeating the above words, while he was really coming down with pneumonia. Next day, when his friends were asked about him, they said: "Yes, some one was saying something good about him yesterday, and now we are afraid we are going to lose him."

According to a Natchez informant, sneezing when eating meant that one would hear of a death; also that someone was talking about him. If one sneezed when he had pneumonia it was a sign he would get well.

When it began to rain after a dry spell the old Creeks would not take things in under cover too hurriedly lest the rain should stop.

---

[90] For some further light on this subject see the section on burial customs, pp. 388–398 in the preceding paper.

[91] Bartram, Trans. Am. Eth. Soc., vol. III, p. 27.

If the bodies of young children were not put into trees in the way elsewhere described it was thought there would be a drought.[93] If, after they had been so disposed of, it began to get dry, the people would go to the tree where the body had been placed and sprinkle water all about it.

That locations might be considered lucky was shown in the case of my Alabama interpreter. After he had lost two wives in succession the people said that something about the situation of his house was "wrong," so he changed it.

An Indian preacher, who, of course, was glad to see Biblical resemblances in native lore, told me that there was a story of a great and long-continued drought in which the people were fed on bread and meat by The One Above. This bread is said to have been "something like white peas" (lady peas).

The annual busk was the principal occasion with them. Bartram observed in one town that they kept Sunday in his time out of respect to the white people,[94] but this custom could never have been very widespread.

SACRIFICES

Sacrifices or offerings similar in kind were made by all of the southern Indians. Adair says:

"They sacrifice in the woods, the milt, or a large fat piece of the first buck they kill, both in their summer and winter hunt; and frequently the whole carcass. This they offer up, either as a thanksgiving for the recovery of health and for their former success in hunting; or that the divine care and goodness may be still continued to them. . . . Formerly, every hunter observed the very same religious economy; but now it is practised only by those who are the most retentive of their old religious mysteries. . .

"The Muskohge Indians sacrifice a piece of every deer they kill at their hunting camps, or near home; if the latter, they dip their middle finger in the broth, and sprinkle it over the domestic tombs of their dead, to keep them out of the power of evil spirits, according to their mythology. . .

"The common sort of Indians, in these corrupt times, only sacrifice a small piece of unsalted fat meat, when they are rejoicing in their divine presence, singing Yo Yo, etc. for their success and safety [in case they have lost none of their companions]: but . . . both the war-leader and his religious assistant go into the woods as soon as they are purified, and there sacrifice the first deer they kill. . .

"They who sacrifice in the woods, do it only on the particular occasions now mentioned; unless incited by a dream, which they esteem a monitory lesson of the Deity." [95]

---

[93] See p. 393.   [94] Bartram, Travels, pp 455–456.   [95] Adair, Hist. Am. Inds., pp. 117–119.

Elsewhere he states that "when in the woods, the Indians cut a small piece out of the lower part of the thighs of the deer they kill, length-ways and pretty deep. Among the great number of venison-hams they bring to our trading houses, I do not remember to have observed one without it."[96] Again "the Indian women always throw a small piece of the fattest of the meat into the fire when they are eating, and frequently before they begin to eat. Sometimes they view it with a pleasing attention, and pretend to draw omens from it. They firmly believe such a method to be a great means of producing temporal good things, and of averting those that are evil.[97] He was informed by those whites who had become used to living in the Indian manner "that the Indian men observe the daily sacrifice both at home, and in the woods, with new-killed venison; but that otherwise they decline it."[97]

Of course most of these are merely taboos connected with the hunting of deer. Pope says on this point:

"The *Creeks* regularly make a Burnt Offering of what they conceive to be the most delicious Parts of every Animal taken in Hunting, before they presume to taste a Mouthful. The Parts they commit to the Flames are proportioned to the Size of the Animal, probably about 2 or 3 lb. from a *Buffalo*, and still less in a regular gradation down to the smallest Quadrupede, Fish or Bird."[98]

I have no confirmation or contradiction of the gradations of sacrifice here mentioned, but it is well known even to the living Indians that the old people used to put a little food into the fire before eating. The same thing is noticed in Adair's account of the Creek who railed upon the fire for burning him after the good treatment he had given it.[99] One of my informants had seen the Nuyaka Indians "feed the fire" with turkey during their fall festivities accompanied by hunting and ball games.

TABOOS

The religion of these people, and, as we shall presently see, their medicine, was seamed through and through with the idea that similarity in appearance means similarity in nature, that similarity in one property involves similarity in all the other properties, and that association of any kind will result in communicating properties from one thing or person to another. This is particularly true about things which are taken into the system by eating and drinking, but applies in other ways as well. Adair says on this point:

"They believe that nature is possest of such a property, as to transfuse into men and animals the qualities, either of the food they use, or of those objects that are presented to their senses; he who

96 Adair, Hist. Am. Inds., pp. 137–138.   98 Pope, Tour, p. 59.
97 Ibid., p. 115.   99 See p. 484.

feeds on venison, is according to their physical system, swifter and
more sagacious than the man who lives on the flesh of the clumsy
bear, or helpless dunghill fowls, the slow-footed tame cattle, or the
heavy wallowing swine. This is the reason that several of their old
men recommend, and say, that formerly their greatest chieftains
observed a constant rule in their diet, and seldom ate of any animal
of a gross quality, or heavy motion of body, fancying it conveyed
a dulness through the whole system, and disabled them from exerting
themselves with proper vigor in their martial, civil, and religious
duties." [1]

A little farther on he tells us that it was customary in all the Indian
tribes to eat the heart of a slain enemy "in order to inspire them with
courage." He had seen some of their warriors drink out of a human
skull in order to "imbibe the good qualities it formerly contained." [2]

This idea is one of the cardinal principles on which their medicine is
built and was shared by every tribe in America that has been investi-
gated. Adair introduces it in order to draw a parallel between the
taboos of the Israelites and those of the Indians, but most of the
Indian instances which he cites are to be accounted for in the way
explained by him above or because it was believed that the animal
in question would bring on a certain disease, a matter to be elaborated
presently. Nevertheless it is worth while to take note of the things
from which they abstained in his time, even though we fail to discover
in that traces of a Jewish origin. He says that they refused to eat all
birds of prey and birds of night, and a little farther on he mentions
specifically eagles, ravens, crows, buzzards, swallows, bats, and every
species of owl. He also adds flies, mosquitoes, and gnats. They did
not eat many carnivorous animals or such as lived on nasty food, as
hogs, wolves, panthers, foxes, cats, mice, rats. All beasts of prey except
the bear were "unhallowed"—also all amphibious quadrupeds, horses,
fowls, moles, the opossum, and all kinds of reptiles. [3] He says that
the old traders could remember when they first began to eat beaver. [4]

Hogs and domestic fowls were probably tabooed at first because
strange to the Indians and in the case of the hog because it is a heavy,
awkward looking animal and might communicate such properties to
the eater.

"When swine were first brought among them, they deemed it such
a horrid abomination in any of their people to eat that filthy and
impure food, that they excluded the criminal from all religious com-
munion in their circular town-house, or in their quadrangular holy
ground at the annual expiation of sins, equally as if he had eaten
unsanctified fruits. After the yearly atonement was made at the
temple, he was indeed re-admitted to his usual privileges." [5]

[1] Adair, Hist. Am. Inds., p. 133.   [4] Ibid., p. 132.
[2] Ibid., p. 135.   [5] Ibid., p. 133.
[3] Ibid., pp. 130–138.

From want of any independent information on this point this must be left without comment. Of course, Adair is anxious to make the most of such a taboo in his desire to establish a Hebrew origin for his red friends, and this is naturally extended to the opossum, after which the Indians named the hog. Still, what he says may be true, that "several of the old Indians assure us, they formerly reckoned it as filthy uneatable an animal, as a hog." [6] The instances which Adair gives in proof of the existence of these taboos all tend to prove that they abstained from them generally for fear of some disease or limitation which the animal might communicate. He says that they abstained from swallowing flies, mosquitoes, or gnats because they believed that they bred sickness or worms, "according to the quantity that goes into them." [7] Upon one occasion Adair shot a small fat hawk which he strongly importuned an old woman to take and dress, but although there was no meat of any kind in camp, "she, as earnestly refused it for fear of contracting pollution, which she called the 'accursed sickness,' supposing disease would be the necessary effect of such an impurity." [8] Again he says that "they abhor moles so exceedingly that they will not allow their children even to touch them for fear of hurting their eye-sight; reckoning it contagious." [9]

Other food taboos mentioned by Adair are against eating an animal that had died of itself, a young animal newly weaned, and blood. The first of these may be commended as a taboo of real medicinal value and the reason given by themselves, that the animal might have died of a contagious disease, is just as valid to-day. Adair has the following to say regarding this taboo.

"None of them will eat any animal whatsoever, if they either know, or suspect that it died of itself. I lately asked one of the women the reason of throwing a dung-hill-fowl out of doors, on the cornhouse; she said, that she was afraid, *Oophe Abeeka Hakset Illeh*,[9a] 'it died with the distemper of the mad dogs,' and that if she had eaten it, it would have afflicted her in the very same manner. I said, if so, she did well to save herself from danger, but at the same time, it seemed she had forgotten the cats. She replied, 'that such impure animals would not contract the accursed sickness, on account of any evil thing they eat; but that the people who ate of the flesh of the swine that fed on such polluting food, would certainly become mad.'

"In the year 1766, a madness seized the wild beasts in the remote woods of West-Florida, and about the same time the domestic dogs were attacked with the like distemper; the deer were equally infected. The Indians in their winter's hunt, found several lying dead, some in a helpless condition, and others fierce and mad. But though they

---

[6] Adair, Hist. Am. Inds., p. 16.
[7] Ibid., p. 131.
[8] Ibid., pp. 130–131.

[9] Ibid., p. 133.
[9a] *Ofi abeka haksit illih.*

are all fond of increasing their number of deer-skins, both from emulation and for profit, yet none of them durst venture to flay them, lest they should pollute themselves, and thereby incur bodily evils. The headman of the camp told me, he cautioned one of the *Hottuk Hakse,* who had resided a long time at Savannah, from touching such deer, saying to him *Chehaksinna,* 'Do not become vicious and mad,' for *Isse Hakset Illehtàhah,* 'the deer were mad, and are dead'; adding, that if he acted the part of *Hakse,* he would cause both himself, and the rest of the hunting camp to be spoiled; nevertheless he shut his ears against his honest speech, and brought those dangerous deerskins to camp. But the people would not afterward associate with him; and he soon paid dear for being *Hakse,* by a sharp splintered root of a cane running almost through his foot, near the very place where he first polluted himself; and he was afraid some worse ill was still in wait for him." [10]

Adair is also very insistent regarding the blood taboo, and cites the case of a woman who believed "she had *Abeeka Ookproo,* 'the accursed sickness,' because she had eaten a great many fowls after the manner of the white people, with the *Issish Ookproo,* 'accursed blood,' in them." Afterwards she would never eat fowls unless they had been bled to death. [11] This must also be left unverified. While there was probably truth in it it is doubtful whether it had the importance attributed to it by Adair, who is again anxious to make a point for his Hebrew theory. The taboo against eating a newly weaned animal is probably correct, since one kind of disease was traced to such an animal in later times, as we shall presently see. Adair says that the old men not merely refrained from eating it but thought "they would suffer damage, even by the bare contact." [12] He also cites instances of Indians refusing to eat with the traders for fear of pollution, [13] but this was less on account of the whites themselves than what might be contained in their dishes. Taboos were so numerous with the old time Indians that parallels with the taboos of any other nation could be found without a great deal of difficulty.

A few miscellaneous beliefs bearing upon taboos may be added, obtained principally from the Natchez doctor so frequently quoted.

If a hunter ate the head of a turkey, gnats and similar flying insects would come about him so closely and in such numbers as to interfere with his vision.

If he ate the tail of a deer the deer would become wild and the hunter could not approach them.

Nothing half cooked and nothing young was to be eaten, nor should one wash his face with soap or bathe in warm water. On

[10] Adair, Hist. Am. Inds., pp. 131–132. Chickasaw words: *hàtàk haksi; chihaksina; isi haksit illitoha.*
[11] Ibid., p. 135. Chickasaw words: *abeka okpulo; issish okpulo.*
[12] Ibid., p. 136.
[13] Ibid., pp. 133–134.

the contrary he must go to cold running water in the morning, even though it were covered with ice, and, breaking the ice, if necessary, plunge into that. He must go in when daylight first showed itself and remain until the sun was up.[13a] This, of course, applies to the baths universally taken in the Southeast every morning and may be overdrawn in details.[14]

An individual taboo of my informant, or means of obtaining luck, was to drink from a cup held in his right hand while he faced the east.

The Natchez and Cherokee ate their food cold, believing it was better for their teeth.

Breaking wind was associated with manliness.

Among the Creeks I was told that when a story-teller finished his narrative he would spit, and then another would have to contribute a story in return, and in this way the cue was taken up by one after another "until the children went to bed."

MUSIC AND DANCING[14a]

Their musical instruments were the drum, rattle, and a kind of flute. Adair makes mention of a stringed instrument, and the mere notice of this would be important if we could prove that it was truly aboriginal. Pope speaks of the Indians in his time dancing for several hours to the music of the violin; but if so, this was a late innovation. The flute was used only by individuals and was never employed in ceremonies, as was constantly the case with the drum and rattle. The Alabama flute was made of two pieces of cedar hollowed out and fastened together with buckskin. There were six holes along the sides toward one end and on top toward the other was placed a separate piece of cedar covering two additional holes. All were bound with buckskin at frequent intervals. Flutes were sometimes made of cane. It may be said of the drum and rattle that the one was an almost invariable and the latter a very frequent accompaniment of their dances.

The drum was made by sawing off a cypress knee close to the ground and stretching a buckskin over the wide end (pl. 13, a). This buckskin was wet from time to time to make it sound properly. Anciently an earthen pot was also employed, and in later times they resorted to a keg partly filled with water and covered with buckskin or cowhide. The rattle was made of a gourd containing 30 or 40 small pebbles, with a stick about a foot long run through it as a handle. In later times a coconut was substituted for the gourd. The chief of the Mikasuki remembered to have heard of still another kind of

[13a] Or as another informant expressed it, "from the second call of the crow until sun up."
[14] See pp. 365-366.
[14a] The interested reader should consult "Ceremonial Songs of the Creek and Yuchi Indians," by Frank G. Speck, in Anthropological Publications of the Museum of the University of Pennsylvania, vol. I, no. 2, Philadelphia, 1911.

rattle as being in use in old times. It was said to be large and flat, but he had never seen one. Very likely it was the turtle-shell rattle, for we know that such a rattle was employed. The women dancers, or rather the leaders among them, as we know, had several tortoise-shell rattles fastened to their calves. Neither the drum nor the rattle was painted. An experienced man or woman acted as leader, and sometimes there were two or more. The usual circuit was sinistral, and this was departed from only to introduce variety. One reason given for the accustomed circuit is that the dancers carried feather fans in their left hands to screen their eyes from the fire while their right hands, the more serviceable ones, were left free for any other purpose. Another reason was that the sun goes that way, for in almost everything observance of the signs of the sun and moon are in evidence. Purely social dances were held most often, it is said, when the moon was full, but ceremonies were performed near the period of the new moon. The fact that dances were held so often in the full of the moon, however, gave early travelers an impression that the Indians observed a ceremony every month. While there were, as we shall note presently, certain ceremonies observed from time to time, most of those that have passed as such were little more than social dances. Although nearly all Indians were intensely fond of dancing, I was told that some persons did not like to dance because they thought dancing would hurt their bones. On the other hand there was a saying among the Creeks that they had to dance after taking medicine in order to overcome it. Otherwise they thought it would get the better of and kill them.

Regarding their songs and dances Bartram remarks as follows:

"They have an endless variety of steps, but the most common, and that which I term the most civil, and indeed the most admired and practised amongst themselves, is a slow shuffling alternate step; both feet move forward one after the other, first the right foot foremost, and next the left, moving one after the other, in opposite circles, i. e. first a circle of young men, and within, a circle of young women, moving together opposite ways, the men with the course of the sun, and the females contrary to it; the men strike their arm with the open hand, and the girls clap hands, and raise their shrill sweet voices, answering an elevated shout of the men at stated times of termination of the stanzas; and the girls perform an interlude or chorus separately.

"To accompany their dances they have songs of different classes, as martial, bacchanalian and amorous; which last, I must confess, are extravagantly libidinous; and they have moral songs, which seem to be the most esteemed and practised, and answer the purpose of religious lectures.

"Some of their most favourite songs and dances, they have from their enemies, the Chactaws; for it seems these people are very eminent for poetry and music; every town amongst them strives to excel each other in composing new songs for dances; and by a custom amongst them, they must give at least one new song, for exhibition, at every annual busk." [15]

The last paragraph records an important tendency observed in many other parts of America, and in this case we have it confirmed by personal observation, for a few days after the arrival of Bartram at Muklasa town a youth in his party who had spent some time in the Choctaw country communicated to the townspeople at their earnest solicitation certain of the songs he had learned.[16]

Swan says:

"In general, their dances are performed with the most violent contortions of the limbs, and an excessive exertion of the muscular powers.

"They have sometimes most farcial dramatic representations, which terminate in the grossest obscenity." [17]

The dances peculiar to the busk will be considered in connection with that ceremonial. The others were principally animal dances, some of which were danced at the time of the busk and some not. Jackson Lewis gave me the following names of dances:

Tcołáko obánga, "the horse dance."

Totolos obánga, "the chicken dance."

Yanása obánga, "the bison dance."

Okiánwa obánga, "the catfish dance."

Futco obánga, "the duck dance."

Akátáláswá obánga, "the small frog dance" (the akátáláswa is a small and very nòisy frog).

Isábá obánga, "the garfish dance."

Yábifega obánga, "the sheep dance."

Yifolo obánga, "the screech-owl dance."

Tcula obánga, "the fox dance."

Istikini obánga, "the horned-owl dance."

Itchas obánga, "the beaver dance."

Kowegi obánga, "the quail dance."

Hitute obánga, "the snow dance."

Kono obánga, "the skunk dance."

Tcito obánga, "the snake dance."

Wátolá obánga, "the crane dance."

Nokos obánga, "the bear dance."

Ogiyīha obánga, "the mosquito dance."

Suli obánga, "the buzzard dance."

Atculálgi obánga, "old people's dance."

[15] Bartram, Travels, pp. 503–504.
[16] Ibid., p. 505.
[17] Schoolcraft, Ind. Tribes, vol. V, p 277.

Poko imobánga, "the ball dance." (I presume this was danced in connection with the ball games.)

My most complete list was from the Alabama in Texas and was as follows:

Tcitcoba bitka, "the horse dance."
Nita bitka, "the bear dance."
Yanasa bitka, "the bison dance."
Kono bitka, "the skunk dance."
Tcoskáni bitka, "the duck dance."
Tcola bitka, "the fox dance."
Tcintcuba bitka, "the alligator dance."
Kitíni bitka, "the horned-owl dance."
Ōfolō bitka, "the screech-owl dance."
Akága bitka, "the chicken dance."
Tcofkoni bitka, "the bone dance."
Wokaskila bitka, "the tree-frog dance."
Łáło bitka, "the fish dance."
Isbák tokolo bitka, "the double-headed dance."
Páspa bitka, "the bread dance."
Sátáne bitka, "the wood-tick dance."
Sinte bitka, "the snake dance."
Sátá bitka, "the terrapin dance."
Okadjibándja bitka, "the parroquet (?) dance."
Itibitilga bitka, "the war dance."
Oktcál'ā bitka, "the blackbird dance."
Kowegi bitka, "the quail dance."
Tcukfi bitka, "the rabbit dance."
Tcokce bitka, "the pumpkin dance" (a very old dance).
Iteheci bitka, "the friends' dance."
Pátka bitka, "the bed dance."
Bitka atcōba, "the old dance."
Taske bitka, "the scalp dance."
Akita bitka, "the ākita dance."
Kinia bitka, "the kinia dance."

The aged chief of the Mikasuki knew of the horse, chicken, quail, skunk, old man's, duck, garfish, alligator, terrapin, crow, corn, hair, and chigoe dances, the last four of which do not occur in the other lists. David Cummings knew of cow and wolf dances, and Zach Cook of leaf and hináta dances. My most complete account of the native dances being from the Alabama, the following descriptions will be based upon them.

When they dressed for the dances the Alabama men frequently painted a large red spot on each cheek and a red line down the nose. The women put a smaller red spot on each cheek and omitted the ine. Occasionally yellow was used instead of red, and in the times of which my informant had any remembrance the paints were obtained from stores. Charcoal was used to blacken the upper lip.

These colors were for appearance only; they had no religious or other significance. The silver crowns and the pouches hung at the side and fastened by straps over the opposite shoulder were worn only at dances, except that the last were taken when traveling or going to town. New buckskin leggings were also worn at dances, but the handkerchief turbans were worn all of the time. The silver gorgets were generally assumed only for dances, but occasionally old ones were carried about at all times. While the hair was always made into four braids the beaded ornaments at the ends were for festivals or when the owner was going to town.

Two of these dances, the horned-owl dance and the snake dance, were never performed by the Alabama in June, July, or August, because in both they followed a serpentine course like that of a snake and people feared that those reptiles would be offended with them and bite them. The horned-owl dance is said to have been danced only in September. Every night, after these dances were over, the participants put their feet up to the fire so that the snakes could not see to bite them, and they warmed their hands and rubbed their eyes with them so that they themselves could see the snakes easily and would not step on them. The snake dance was danced a long time ago. All that I can add regarding it is Jackson Lewis's statement that it was danced entirely by women, and an implication on the part of Swan that the leader of this dance carried a wooden snake in his hands, but what Lewis said does not seem to be in agreement with what my Alabama informant had heard.

The horned-owl dance was evidently a greater favorite and was danced more frequently, and it was connected with those feasts to which reference has already been made. To summon people to this dance a man went around on horseback—sometimes accompanied by a second—carrying in his hands a peculiar baton. This was made of a cane about 12 feet long, at the outer end of which was a hoop made of hickory, white oak, or some other suitable wood. About five deer tails, and sometimes a loaf of bread, were fastened to this. Bearing it, he visited every house to make the announcement.

The horned-owl dance was always in September. There was no drummer but one old man walked about perhaps 10 feet from the fire shaking a rattle and singing, while the men and women danced around the fire inside sinistrally. The rattler was also song leader; the men sang with him but the women did not sing. There was no definite order in which the men and women danced, except that one man did not immediately follow another. Each man held a handkerchief by one corner and a woman following held the opposite corner of the handkerchief. If another woman, or other women, danced beside her, they held her by the elbows. The dancers were

led by a second old man, and all of the men carried turkey-tail fans.
They danced for a while sinistrally, and then turned around and
danced dextrally. When they were through the women remained
standing in a row southeast of the fire. Then the old man took the
baton already mentioned, stood opposite them and let the hoop
fall on the head of each woman in succession, saying as he did so,
"pátcicpălō', make bread." This was because the women were to
make bread while the men were off hunting. Another old man
stood beside the first and counted the women off, "one, two, three,"
etc., and when he made the last count all of the men said "Ŏh"
in a very high-pitched voice. Then all the men went after venison,
and at the end of two weeks all brought roast venison to the dancing
ground on the same day. When they were within about half a mile
they discharged their guns and shouted to let it be known that they
were coming. They took the venison to a house at the dance ground
built like a corncrib and laid it down there. That night they began
the horned-owl dance again, and after it was over the men sat down
on sheepskins, bearskins, or blankets all around the fire. Then the
women came with dishes of bread and set them down by the men,
one dish by some, two by others, three or four by others, etc., as
they chose. Two old men now came, each with a kolbe' (a large flat
basket made of cane). They gathered up the bread and redistributed
it to all of the men and boys. Then the old men went to a scaffold
near by and brought a number of sharp sticks already prepared.
They laid one of these by every man who had received one dish of
bread, two by those who had received two dishes, and so on. Then
the two old men took their kolbes again and brought the venison
which they also distributed. The men took it and put one, two,
three, or more pieces of meat on each stick. Then they held these
up in their hands and each woman got a stick of venison and her dish.
Then the men began to sing while still seated, one man leading with
a rattle. All sang four times and then they stood up and sat down
in their usual places, on logs about 20 paces back from the fire.
They now stood up again and formed a circle surrounding and facing
the women. First the men danced backward, the women following
facing them; then they filed off round the fire in couples, a man
and a woman together. They went around four times and then
went off to one side of the fire, the north for instance, danced inward
in an ever narrowing spiral, turned around and danced out again
in the same way, danced around the fire four times more, and then
danced in a spiral in and out to the west of the fire. In this way they
went all the way round, dancing on the south and east sides also.
Finally they danced four times round the fire. Bread and venison
were given out for four successive nights, and the same dance followed.

SWANTON]   CREEK RELIGION AND MEDICINE   527

This dance was known to Zachariah Cook and William Berryhill
and the latter gave the following account of it which shows that it
was the same thing and was known over the entire Creek country:

The men started out to hunt while the women were making bread.
If the men brought home a deer the first day they gave it to the
women who cooked it and put the flesh into the meat house. That
night they danced, and they did the same thing four days in succession, putting what they killed each day into the meat house. Then
they sacked the bread and meat up, and the women carried the sacks
into the square and danced with them on their backs—though it
was rather hard work. After the dance they handed these sacks to
the male waiters, who distributed them to everyone in the town.
Enough was usually left to supply the visitors among the various
camps—i. e., those who happened to be in the town camping about
the square, not persons especially invited. Then they usually dispersed, eating their food at once or carrying it with them. This
dance was danced just after all the snakes were supposed to have
gone into their holes for the winter. They would not dance it in
summer lest the snakes should bite them. The words of the song
were like this: Dje'hose djehō'se yū'liwå yuhe'å.

Conversely from the custom with regard to the last two, the Alabama avoided dancing the bear dance in winter, for they went
hunting then and they were afraid if they did so a bear would catch
and hurt one of them or one of their dogs. This dance was always
at night, the music being furnished by a drummer and a singer, the
latter without a rattle. The dancers circled about the fire in single
file, men and women alternating and pawing at the air with their
hands in imitation of the bear.

Nearly all of these dances were at night, but the bison dance
was, among the Alabama, always held in the morning before sunrise,
though it could be performed at any time of the year. One man
stood near the fire and furnished the music by beating on a drum
and singing while the participants ran around the fire very rapidly
and at a certain beat of the drum all shouted. This agrees with what
Zachariah Cook says of this dance as seen by him. He states they
went two and two around the fire and at a certain beat came down
together on the ground with both feet. The dance would seem to
have been brought by the Alabama from their old home, for they say
that when they came to east Texas there were no bison there.[18]

---

[18] Schoolcraft, Ind. Tribes, vol. v, p 277. It was made the subject of a painting by Mr J. M. Stanley,
which was one of those destroyed in the Smithsonian fire. He has the following note regarding it: "This
dance is enacted every year during the season of their busk or green-corn dances; and the men, women, and
children all take an active part in the ceremony. They invest themselves with the scalp of the buffalo,
with the horns and tail attached, and dance about in a circle, uttering sounds in imitation of the animal
they represent, with their bodies in a half-bent position, supporting their weight upon their ball-sticks,
which represent the forelegs of the buffalo."—Smithson. Misc. Colls., no. 53, p. 10. He is the only observer
mentioning the participation of children.

With the Mikasuki, the Chiaha, and probably the Creeks generally, the bison dance was held just at sundown of the day of the busk, but while there was still light.[18a] The music was furnished by one drummer and one rattler. At the beginning these two men stood near the ball post and the dancers assembled there, the male dancers each carrying a cane. When all was ready the musicians walked into the yard between the beds and the dancers followed them in couples, two men and two women alternating. Then they danced around the fire until the three songs belonging to this dance, which were rather long, were finished. This dance was followed by the long or old dance.

The fox, ākitä, kinia, and skunk dances are said to have been danced exclusively by women. Jackson Lewis and Cook confirmed this for the Creeks so far as the fox dance is concerned and the chief of the Mikasuki asserted it for the skunk dance. Therefore the custom must have been fairly widespread. At least among the Alabama these dances were always in June, July, or August. Before the fox dance was held two men went all around the grounds to drive the dogs away, for, if any dogs should come in or any men except the two musicians, it would be unlucky. The two musicians, a drummer and a rattler, sat near the fire and they did all of the singing. One of the women acted as leader of the dancers and they went around the fire in sinistral circuit. The dance began slowly and increased in rapidity until it became very fast at the end. The two "dogwhippers" were provided with long sticks with needles, gar teeth, or crawfish claws at the ends, and, if a woman was slow or lazy in dancing, they reached these out and scratched her ankles. Sometimes old women performed this function. My informant himself never saw this, but he has often heard it described. The fox dance may have had some of the other features of the skunk and kinia dances.

The ākitä is said to be a small animal living in the woods and looking like a rat. Charlie Adams, my informant, has never seen one and the creature may be entirely fabulous. During this dance every woman carried in each hand a stick about 2 feet long. On the ends of each stick were four crane feathers of different colors—white, black, blue, etc. The leading woman and the last woman each had entire crane wings on the ends of their sticks. The women would dance around for a certain time sinistrally, and when the singer struck a certain note all turned about, the last woman leading, and danced around dextrally until the note again sounded. They danced twice each way in all.

The kinia is said to be an animal like the ākitä. In this dance the women started around sinistrally, and at certain beats stopped and danced where they were and then at other beats went on again and again stopped. This was repeated about ten times.

The skunk dance was like the kinia, but in this two men came out in front of the file of dancing women holding a stick, one at each end, about 3½ feet from the ground. The women dodged under this one after the other and if one of them touched it, even with her hair ribbons, she, in company with all other women who had touched it, had to cook for all the men and bring the food up to the dance ground. Otherwise the last three dances were like the first.

The chief of the Mikasuki said that the skunk dance took place when peanuts, beans, etc., were ready for gathering—i. e., in September. A drummer and a rattler furnished both instrumental and vocal music for it, but, unlike most dances, in this the women sang in response.

According to Silas Jefferson it took place in October. One man sang the skunk songs while the women danced dressed in men's clothing. They danced four times every night for four nights and on the morning after the last the men went out to drive deer.

From what William McCombs, a Chiaha Indian, has told me of this dance there must, if his memory serves him well, have been considerable variation. He says that this dance was the most sacred of all the animal dances and that for some reason the skunk was considered as chief of all the animals. It was held at the square ground in winter, but without secret ceremonies. A person starting in to dance in this had to keep it up during all four nights. After it was over a great hunt and a great feast took place.

Another dance confined to women was the snow dance, regarding which I have no other information.

The pumpkin and bed dances were danced a long time ago, and my informants knew nothing about them but the names. The same was true of the war and scalp dances.

The blackbird dance is also obsolete, the following reason being given for it. The last time it was performed by the Koasati, whose town was near that of the Alabama, they somehow offended the blackbirds, who bewitched them, causing them to die out. Therefore this is now considered a "wrong dance," and it is used no more.

In the duck dance two men sat on a bench to furnish the music, one drumming and one singing. The dancers formed two files in the following manner: First two men, then two women, then two men, and so on, but the men danced around the fire sinistrally and the women dextrally, the women between the two files of men. Each of the two pairs of men held one end of a handkerchief, and the women passed under it. They danced around the fire four times slowly and four times rapidly, completing the dance. The Mikasuki chief described it in exactly the same way, except he said the dancers danced a minute in front of each other before the women passed under and the men clasped their hands instead of using a handkerchief. They used a rattle but no drum. The men danced dextrally; the women sinistrally. Three songs belonged to it. Cook merely stated that they imitated ducks.

The horse dance was as follows: The music was furnished by two drummers near the fire—or sometimes by only one. They drummed and sang. The men danced in two bands and in single file. The two came from opposite sides of the fire, one from the south, we will say, circling sinistrally outside, and the other, from the north, circling dextrally inside. As the two lines passed the men would kick out at each other like horses. Meantime the women were standing on the outside, each holding a handkerchief by one end, and the second time around each man seized the end of a handkerchief and danced around, the woman following him dancing, until they had danced four times in all. Then all went back to their places and the same thing was repeated three times more, four in all. The Mikasuki horse dance was practically the same except that there was no drummer and but one rattler. There were two songs.

In the alligator dance there was no rattle or drum and no special singers, the men furnishing all of the singing. They danced in one file, men and women alternating, holding the ends of handkerchiefs in front and behind so as to make a continuous string. Although they moved rapidly they arrested their feet in midair for a moment before letting them down, probably imitating the supposed gait of the alligator. There were two songs, repeated indefinitely. This was danced at any time, summer or winter. My informant had seen this twice.

The Mikasuki varied this somewhat. There was one rattler who stood by the fire around which the dancers passed in single file. A man and a woman danced together, the man going backward and holding by both hands the woman, who danced forward. At a certain turn in the music they reversed their positions, the woman dancing backward and the man forward. There were about seven songs to this dance.

The screech-owl dance was performed at any time and it was like the alligator dance but there were five or six songs. The songs were like those of the horned-owl dance except that there were over 30 songs for the latter.

In the chicken dance two men sat by the fire, one beating a drum, the other helping him sing. The women came together on the east side of the fire and from there danced all around it once when the drummer struck the drum hard. All the women then went out and each got a man, and brought him in. The partners then clasped hands and danced around the fire, the men going backward first until a certain drumbeat, when they turned around and the women danced backward. There was just one song and they danced until the song had been repeated four times. Then the women assembled at the same place as before, only the men came and got them in their turn; the same thing was repeated four times in all, when they stopped. It was danced at any time, but usually in summer. The Mikasuki had one rattler for this dance and the dancers went around about as in the alligator dance.

In the tree-frog dance there were also two men by the fire singing, one beating on a drum. The dancers were in two files, two men alternating with two women. When the drummer beat the drum all of the men squatted down on their haunches, the woman remaining standing. Then the two singers and the squatting men all sang a song. At a certain beat of the drum all stopped singing and began dancing around again. They danced around the fire four times and stopped, and the men squatted down once more. The whole was repeated four times. It was danced at any season.

The bone dance was danced at night at any time of the year and it was very fast, "like a nigger dance." Because it was so fast some women did not like to participate in it. One man beat the drum and sang. The dancers were in couples, a man and a woman side by side, holding hands. They danced forward for a while and at a certain beat turned round and danced backward, at another beat danced forward, and so on. They went around the fire four times. There were two songs, one sung while they were standing still, another while they were dancing.

The dance often spoken of as "the fish dance" (Làlo obánga, in Creek) is identical with the garfish dance, although, as we have seen, there was a catfish dance. Among the Alabama the garfish dance was said to be just like the chicken dance, only faster. There was one drummer and one person to help him sing, and there were eight songs. According to the Mikasuki chief it was almost the same as the alligator dance except that the songs were shorter. This dance seems to have been in especial favor with the Koasati, and according to one informant the garfish was their tribal mark. It would seem from the account of it, however, that the Koasati garfish dance was either a distinct dance or very much modified. David Cummings, who passed his early youth with the old Koasati, had the following to say about it:

In the fall, September or October, the men went out hunting and stayed out about a month. When they got near home on their return they uttered whoops, and when the women heard that they said, "The hunters are coming home with deer meat and turkeys." After that they appointed a day on which to dance the fish dance. Every man who danced this had a stick made like a garfish, its mouth being open and a piece of cedar placed in it. About a dozen men were invited to take part in this dance, word being sent to them by two ta'palas.

They formed a complete circle under the arbor which covered the Koasati square and, holding the wooden fish in their hands, jumped up and down and danced. The musicians sat in the chiefs' bed. At a certain time in the song all of the dancers said "yū+ē" and all changed places, each moving to the station vacated by the man next in front of him. In this manner they moved about the entire circle. Except for the above exclamation the singing was all done by the musicians in the chiefs' bed. Afterwards there was a great feast (hompila), consisting of all sorts of cooked foods, everybody being invited into the square ground. Then they danced the common or stomp dance all that night, and everyone was compelled to attend, the old women and children being the only persons exempted.

William McCombs stated that in the garfish dance, as he knew it, the participants grouped themselves together in four circles at each of the four corners of the square in succession, beginning at the southeast and passing in the usual direction. This appears to have been like the Koasati dance just described, as was probably the fish dance mentioned by Swan in which the leader, male or female, carried a wooden fish.[19]

In the double-headed dance, there was one drummer and one other person to help him sing. There were two parties of dancers and a leader for each, which went round the fire in opposite directions, one outside of the other. After they had gone round four times the leaders took each other by the hand and all of their followers did the same, and they danced backward and forward a few times, away from and toward the fire. Then they let go and danced around the fire in the same manner four times more. After dancing backward and forward for the fourth time all shouted and stopped. There were two songs.

When the quail dance was to be undertaken one man sat close to the ball posts away from the fire beating a drum and all of the men and women danced around him. The men and women alternated and walked like quails. There were two songs and they made four circuits during each. This was danced at night and sometimes just before a ball game. The Mikasuki used a rattler instead of a drummer and he stood close by the fire. The dancers went by couples, a man and a woman holding each other's hands. There were four songs.

In the terrapin dance a drummer and an assistant singer sat by the fire to furnish the music. The dancers went in single file, men and women alternating. Each dancer clasped both hands together and moved them about to right and left, jumping a little at times. The leaders kept repeating "kwi'" over and over and the rest of the dancers said "haha." There was only one song, and they stopped

[19] Schoolcraft, Ind. Tribes, vol. v, p 277.

after they had danced around four times. According to the Mikasuki chief the dancers went in double file, men and women alternating but not holding each other's hands. One rattler furnished the music and there were four songs.

In the tick dance no drum was used and there were no special singers, the men doing all the singing. They went in single file, men and women alternating, and holding the ends of handkerchiefs to make a continuous line. They assumed a kind of staggering step. There were 10 songs and when the last was sung they raised a shout and stopped. This might be danced at any time.

The Okádjibándja dance was almost the same as the tick dance. It was danced by men and women in two files side by side. All of the men were outside and all of the women inside. The men and women held each other's hands and all went around the fire with an undulating motion, sometimes near the fire and sometimes removed from the fire. There were two songs. They danced eight times and then stopped. The men all sang; there was no other music. It was danced at any time.

In the rabbit dance there was no drummer, only one man with a rattle who was assisted in singing by all of the other men. There were three songs. The dancers were arranged in couples, a man and a woman, the women all being inside, with one old woman acting as leader. They danced around the fire four times and then stopped. They went faster and faster until some fell down. After they had gone round the fire twice more they went out to one side as in the horned-owl dance, then round the fire twice more, out at another side, round the fire again, and so on until they had been to all four sides. They sang the first song while standing still, the second song while going round the fire, and the third song while circling at the side of the fire.

In the friends' dance one man sitting on a bench near the fire drummed and was assisted in singing by a second man. When they began singing two men came in, walked all the way round the fire, went out again, and brought in two women. The four walked around the fire, a man and a woman side by side, and then the two women went out and brought in two more men. They went around again when the two last men went for two more women. This was kept up until all were brought in. After they were thus made friends the women danced around inside and the men outside about four times and then all stopped. There were two songs, one sung after all had been brought in. This could be danced at any time.

The following dances were described by the Mikasuki chief, but were unknown to, or forgotten by, the Alabama.

In the crow dance they went around in two files, first two women, then two men, and so on. At a certain time in the dance the women turned around and danced backward facing the two men and then turned back again. There were two songs; a rattle only was used.

In the corn dance they went in two files, a man and a woman side by side. The rattle was used alone and there were six songs.

In the hair dance two women went together and then two men alternately. There were four songs and the rattle only was used.

In the chigoe dance men and women mingled, joined hands, and danced round the fire in single file. A rattle was used and one song.

The old men's dance was danced about the time when pokeweed berries are ripe—i. e., about the middle of October. Young men were usually the performers. They fixed themselves up in imitation of old-time Indians. Each wore a mask made out of a pumpkin, gourd, or melon, holes being cut for the eyes and mouth and the latter provided with teeth made out of grains of corn. A headgear was constructed out of leaf stalks of the sumac, the small ends of which were tied together and the body opened out and fitted over the head. Long earrings were fastened to the mask and a shawl thrown over the head behind. They stained the outside of the mask with the berries of the pokeweed (osá in Creek). Finally the performer fastened tortoise-shell rattles on his legs, drew a blanket round himself, and performed all sorts of antics to make people laugh. He carried a bow and arrows improvised for the occasion, pretended to see game, and did other things supposed to be amusing. The children were scared half to death with his performances and William Berryhill, one of my informants, well remembers how frightened he was at them. The dance was known also to the most of my other old informants.[19a]

Regarding the catfish, small frog, sheep, beaver, cow, crane, and wolf dances I have no information other than that they existed. In the mosquito dance the women played jokes on the male dancers by pricking them with pins. The buzzard dance is said to have been a very pretty affair, the arms of the dancers being spread out and made to flap like the wings of buzzards.

The drunken dance was used just before gatherings broke up. The people formed a circle, acted as if they were intoxicated, and gradually scattered backward into the bushes and disappeared. It is said to have been like the skunk dance.

CEREMONIES

MISCELLANEOUS CEREMONIES

In the section on music and dancing I have spoken of the monthly ceremonies which early writers, including Bartram and Du Pratz, allege were performed by the southern Indians. This may be explained partly on the ground that social dances took place oftenest near the full of the moon. But, while most of the dances and feasts which I have described elsewhere can be explained as furnishing

[19a] See p. 556.

outlets for the purely social instincts, ceremonial elements entered
into certain of them in such a way that it might be difficult to say
where the social element ended and the ceremonial element began.
There is a suggestion of this sort in the regulations connected with
the snake, horned-owl, and skunk dances.   Ceremonies or fasts of a
somewhat extemporaneous character were undertaken from time to
time in cases of national distress, as we learn from Bartram, who says:

"At this time the town [Atasi] was fasting, taking medicine, and
I think I may say praying, to avert a grievous calamity of sickness,
which had lately afflicted them, and laid in the grave abundance of
their citizens.   They fast seven or eight days, during which time they
eat or drink nothing but a meagre gruel, made of a little cornflour and
water; taking at the same time by way of medicine or physic, a strong
decoction of the roots of the Iris versicolor, which is a powerful
cathartic." [20]

Religious ceremony was more or less mixed up with social relaxation in the feasts held after a successful hunt or upon the arrival of
strangers.   Bartram again gives us a view of one of these impromptu
gatherings which he witnessed in the Seminole town of Talahasutci,
of which a man called by the whites the White King was then miko.

"On our arrival at the trading house, our chief was visited by the
head men of the town, when instantly the White King's arrival in
town was announced: a messenger had before been sent in to prepare
a feast, the king and his retinue having killed several bears.   A fire
was now kindled in the area of the public square; the royal standard
was displayed, and the drum beat to give notice to the town of the
royal feast.

"The ribs and the choice pieces of the three great fat bears already
well barbecued or broiled, were brought to the banqueting house in
the square, with hot bread; and honeyed water for drink.

"When the feast was over in the square (where only the chiefs
and warriors were admitted, with the white people), the chief priest,
attended by slaves, came with baskets and carried off the remainder
of the victuals, etc. which was distributed amongst the families of
the town.   The king then withdrew, repairing to the council-house
in the square, whither the chiefs and warriors, old and young, and
such of the whites as chose, repaired also; the king, war chief, and
several ancient chiefs and warriors were seated on the royal cabins;
the rest of the head men and warriors, old and young, sat on the cabins
on the right hand of the king's: the cabins or seats on the left, and
on the same elevation, are always assigned for the white people,
Indians of other towns, and such of their own people as choose.

"Our chief, with the rest of the white people in town, took their
seats according to order: tobacco and pipes were brought; the calu-

[20] Bartram, Travels, p. 454.

met was lighted and smoked, circulating according to the usual forms
and ceremony; and afterwards black drink concluded the feast.
The king conversed, drank cassine, and associated familiarly with
his people and with us.

"After the public entertainment was over, the young people began
their music and dancing in the square, whither the young of both
sexes repaired, as well as the old and middle aged: this frolick continued all night."[21]

Bartram has the following regarding the ceremonies connected
with an ordinary Creek council:

"As their virgils and manner of conducting their vespers and mys-
tical fire in this rotunda [the tcokofa], are extremely singular, and
altogether different from the customs and usages of any other people,
I shall proceed to describe them. In the first place, the governor or
officer who has the management of this business, with his servants
attending, orders the black drink to be brewed, which is a decoction
or infusion of the leaves and tender shoots of the Cassine: this is
done under an open shed or pavilion, at twenty or thirty yards distance, directly opposite the door of the council-house. Next he
orders bundles of dry canes to be brought in: these are previously
split and broken in pieces to about the length of two feet, and then
placed obliquely crossways upon one another on the floor, forming a
spiral circle round about the great centre pillar, rising to a foot or
eighteen inches in height from the ground; and this circle spreading
as it proceeds round and round, often repeated from right to left,
every revolution encreases its diameter, and at length extends to
the distance of ten or twelve feet from the centre, more or less, according to the length of time the assembly or meeting is to continue.
By the time these preparations are accomplished, it is night, and the
assembly have taken their seats in order. The exterior extremity or
outer end of the spiral circle takes fire and immediately rises into a
bright flame (but how this is effected I did not plainly apprehend;
I saw no person set fire to it; there might have been fire left on the
earth, however I neither saw nor smelt fire or smoke until the blaze
instantly ascended upwards), which gradually and slowly creeps
round the centre pillar, with the course of the sun, feeding on the
dry canes, and affords a cheerful, gentle and sufficient light until the
circle is consumed, when the council breaks up. Soon after this
illumination takes place, the aged chiefs and warriors are seated on
their cabins or sophas on the side of the house opposite the door,
in three classes or ranks, rising a little, one above or behind the other;
and the white people and red people of confederate towns in the
like order on the left hand; a transverse range of pillars, supporting
a thin clay wall about breast high, separating them: the king's

21 Bartram, Travels, pp. 233-235.

cabin or seat is in front; the next to the back of it the head warriors; and the third or last accommodates the young warriors, etc. The great war chief's seat or place is on the same cabin with, and immediately to the left hand of the king, and next to the white people; and to the right hand of the mico or king the most venerable head-men and warriors are seated.

"The assembly being now seated in order, and the house illuminated, two middle aged men, who perform the office of slaves or servants, pro tempore, come in together at the door, each having very large conch shells full of black drink, and advance, with slow, uniform and steady steps, their eyes or countenances lifted up, singing very low but sweetly; they come within six or eight paces of the king's and white people's cabins, when they stop together, and each rests his shell on a tripos or little table, but presently takes it up again, and, bowing very low, advances obsequiously, crossing or interesecting each other about midway: he who rested his shell before the white people now stands before the king, and the other who stopped before the king stands before the white people, and as soon as he raises it to his mouth, the slave utters or sings two notes, each of which continues as long as he has breath; and as long as these notes continue, so long must the person drink or at least keep the shell to his mouth. These two long notes are very solemn, and at once strike the imagination with a religious awe or homage to the Supreme, sounding somewhat like a–hoo—ojah and a–lu—yah.[22] After this manner the whole assembly are treated, as long as the drink and light continue to hold out; and as soon as the drinking begins, tobacco and pipes are brought. The skin of a wild cat or young tyger stuffed with tobacco is brought, and laid at the king's feet, with the great or royal pipe beautifully adorned; the skin is usually of the animals of the king's family or tribe, as the wild-cat, otter, bear, rattle-snake, etc. A skin of tobacco is likewise brought and cast at the feet of the white chief of the town, and from him it passes from one to another to fill their pipes from, though each person has besides his own peculiar skin of tobacco. The king or chief smokes first in the great pipe a few whiffs, blowing it off ceremoniously, first towards the sun, or as it is generally supposed to the Great Spirit, for it is puffed upwards, next towards the four cardinal points, then towards the white people in the house; then the great pipe is taken from the hand of the mico by a slave, and presented to the chief white man, and then to the great war chief, whence it circulates through the rank of head men and warriors, then returns to the king. After this each one fills his pipe from his own or his neighbour's skin."[23]

---

[22] Possibly intended for Yahola and Hayuya (see pp. 485, 544).
[23] Bartram, Travels, pp. 448–452.

By "the royal standard" Bartram means nothing more than the feathered calumet. The drum, as we learn on all hands, was used to call assemblies at the square for whatever purpose, and bear skins were usually laid down for the principal men and their guests on such occasions. The all-night dance mentioned at the end was a familiar accompaniment of the daily lives of the people.

CEREMONY OF THE ASI

At least one ceremony is involved here which was more religious than social and I will proceed to a more intimate account of it. This is the ceremony connected with the taking of the *Ilex vomitoria* or "black drink." The longest and best description of this is given by Swan and is as follows:

"The ceremony of the Black-drink is a military institution, blended with religious opinions.

"The black-drink is a strong decoction of the shrub well known in the Carolinas by the name of Cassina, or the Uupon tea.

"The leaves are collected, parched in a pot until brown, boiled over a fire in the center of the square, dipped out and poured from one pan or cooler into another, and back again, until it ferments and produces a large quantity of white froth, from which, with the purifying qualities the Indians ascribe to it, they style it white-drink; but the liquor of itself, which, if strong, is nearly as black as molasses, is by the white people universally called black-drink.

"It is a gentle diuretic, and, if taken in large quantities, sometimes affects the nerves. If it were qualified with sugar, etc., it could hardly be distinguished in taste from strong bohea tea.

"Except rum, there is no liquor of which the Creek Indians are so excessively fond. In addition to their habitual fondness for it, they have a religious belief that it infallibly possesses the following qualities, viz.: That it purifies them from all sin, and leaves them in a state of perfect innocence; that it inspires them with an invincible prowess in war; and that it is the only solid cement of friendship, benevolence, and hospitality. Most of them really seem to believe that the Great Spirit or Master of breath has communicated the virtues of the black-drink to them, and them only (no other Indians being known to use it as they do),[23a] and that it is a peculiar blessing bestowed on them, his chosen people. Therefore, a stranger going among them can not recommend himself to their protection in any manner so well as by offering to partake of it with them as often as possible.

"The method of serving up black-drink in the square is as follows, viz:

[23a] This was by no means the case since, in one form or another, the drink was used by practically all Southeastern tribes. See below.

" The warriors and chiefs being assembled and seated, three young men acting as masters of ceremony on the occasion, each having a gourd or calabash full of the liquor, place themselves in front of the three greatest chiefs or warriors, and announce that they are ready by the word choh! After a short pause, stooping forward, they run up to the warriors and hold the cup or shell parallel to their mouths; the warriors receive it from them, and wait until the young men fall back and adjust themselves to give what they term the yohullah, or black-drink note. As the young men begin to aspirate the note, the great men place the cups to their mouths, and are obliged to drink during the aspirated note of the young men, which, after exhausting their breath, is repeated on a finer key, until the lungs are no longer inflated. This long aspiration is continued near half a minute, and the cup is taken from the mouth of the warrior who is drinking at the instant the note is finished. The young men then receive the cups from the chiefs or head warriors, and pass them to the others of inferior rank, giving them the word choh! but not the yohullah note. None are entitled to the long black-drink note but the great men, whose abilities and merit are rated on this occasion by the capacity of their stomachs to receive the liquor.

" It is generally served round in this manner three times [24] at every meeting; during the recess of serving it up, they all sit quietly in their several cabins, and amuse themselves by smoking, conversing, exchanging tobacco, etc., and in disgorging what black-drink they have previously swallowed.

" Their mode of disgorging, or spouting out the black-drink, is singular, and has not the most agreeable appearance. After drinking copiously, the warrior, by hugging his arms across his stomach, and leaning forward, disgorges the liquor in a large stream from his mouth, to the distance of six or eight feet. Thus, immediately after drinking, they begin spouting on all sides of the square, and in every direction; and in that country, as well as in others more civilized, it is thought a handsome accomplishment in a young fellow to be able to spout well.

" They come into the square and go out again, on these occasions, without formality." [25]

The following is Adair's account, which shows that the ceremony was almost identical among the Chickasaw:

" There is a species of tea, that grows spontaneously, and in great plenty, along the sea-coast of the two Carolinas, Georgia, and East and West Florida, which we call *Yopon*, or *Cusseena*: the Indians transplant, and are extremely fond of it; they drink it on certain

---

[24] Probably this should be "four times"
[25] Schoolcraft, Ind. Tribes, vol. v, pp. 266–267.

stated occasions, and in their most religious solemnities, with awful invocations; but the women, and children, and those who have not successfully accompanied their holy ark, *pro Aris et Focis*, dare not even enter the sacred square, when they are on this religious duty; otherwise they would be dry-scratched with snakes teeth, fixed in the middle of a split reed, or a piece of wood, without the privilege of warm water to supple the stiffened skin.[25a]

"When this beloved liquid, or supposed holy drink-offering, is fully prepared, and fit to be drank, one of their *Magi* brings two old consecrated conch-shells, out of a place appropriated for containing the holy things, and delivers them into the hands of two religious attendants, who, after a wild ceremony, fill them with the supposed sanctifying, bitter liquid: then they approach near to the two central red and white seats, (which the traders call the war, and beloved cabbins) stooping with their heads and bodies pretty low; advancing a few steps in this posture, they carry their shells with both hands, at an instant, to one of the most principal men on those red and white seats, saying, on a bass key, Yàh, quite short: then, in like manner, they retreat backward, facing each other, with their heads bowing forward, their arms across, rather below their breast, and their eyes half shut; thus, in a very grave, solemn manner, they sing on a strong bass key, the awful monosyllable, O, for the space of a minute: then they strike up majestic He, on the treble, with a very intent voice, as long as their breath allows them; and on a bass key, with a bold voice, and short accent, they at last utter the strong mysterious sound, Wah, and thus finish the great song, or the most solemn invocation of the divine essence . . . The favoured persons, whom the religious attendants are invoking the divine essence to bless, hold the shells with both hands, to their mouths, during the awful sacred invocation, and retain a mouthful of the drink, to spurt out on the ground, as a supposed drink-offering to the great self-existent Giver; which they offer at the end of their draught. If any of the traders, who at those times are invited to drink with them, were to neglect this religious observance, they would reckon us as godless and wild as the wolves of the desert. After the same manner, the supposed holy waters proceed, from the highest to the lowest, in their synedrion: and, when they have ended that awful solemnity, they go round the whole square, or quadrangular place, and collect tobacco from the sanctified sinners, according to ancient custom."[26]

Still another description of this ceremonial is given by Stiggins:

"I shall now enter on their uniform custom of drinking their *āssēe* which is a very strong black tea used by them without any sugar,

---

[25a] See pp. 363–364.
[26] Adair, Hist. Am. Inds., pp. 46–48.

made of eupon or Cassene leaves. Said drink is called by the white men among them the *Black drink*. It is customary at this time and may have been for ages back for the men to meet at their town house or square in every town at least once a week. In the Tuckabatchies, the principal town, they meet every morning to drink their asee, which is prepared for use in the following manner at all places. It is parched first in a large pot of their own manufactory of clay untill the leaves are brown. Then water is applied to the full of the pot and boiled by a man appointed to that service. After boiling, it is cooled in large cooling pans of the same manufactory by one of the oldest chiefs of the town. When it can be poured over his finger without scalding it is cool enough to drink. It is then put into two gourds that would hold near a gallon each with a hole in it of about three quarters of an inch in diameter at which hole they suck it out. Said gourds of assee are very ceremoniously handed round the square to every man by men selected for the purpose and drunk as made, without sugar or any other embellishment. It is singular how this tea operates on them after they drink it, for after they have drunk it they retain it in their stomack for near a half hour. They can discharge their stomack of it as often as they drink it, with seeming ease, spouting it out of their mouth as it were by eructation. After four or five drinks and discharges of their stomack at different times of near a quart at a time, the black drink being over they disperse at or near ten o'clock; it acts as a tonic, as it is drunk of a morning fasting. By the process their stomack is well rinsed and braced up. The taste of the black drink is not disagreeable being not unlike [that of] very strong black tea and nearly of a black colour. No doubt but their custom of drinking the black drink originated through political motives, viz., for the purpose of assembling the towns people frequently at their town house or square in order to keep them united." [27]

A few shorter accounts may be added. The first is by David Taitt:

"I went this morning to the [Tukabahchee] Town hot House where was only a few Old Men sitting and smoking Tobacco. When I went in the men present came a(nd) shook hands with me and offered me their Tobacco to smoke, afterwards they presented me with a Calabash filled with black drink made from the leaves of Casina which they parch in an Earthen pot till they are of a Dark brown Colour, they then put water upon them and boil it up till it is very Strong. They afterwards put a Strainer made of Split Canes into the pot and so take the drink out of the Strenner with a Callabash, entirely free from any leaves, they cool it in a Large Earthen bowle by heaving it up with gourds or Callabashes till

[27] Stiggins, Ms.

they raise a froth on the Top as Strong as that on porter. When it is
Cool enough they fill some gourds with (it) and Carry it into the
hot house in winter or Square in Summer, and present it to the
head man or King of the Town first and likewise to any Stranger
that is present two or three men Singing while the others Drink.
As soon as they have done Singing, they Receive the Callabashes
from head man and Stranger and Exchange them that they may
drink together, then it is handed all round to every person present
without the Ceremony of Singing or Exchanging Cups." [28]

Claiborne incorporates the following in his History of Mississippi:

"When the Creeks meet in council they smoke and have what
they call 'the black drink.' It is made of the leaves of the Cassina
Yapon, a tree resembling the haw-bush. They put the leaves in a
basket and deposit it in a long earthen pot and boil them over a
fire made in the middle of the square under a scaffold. The ceremony
of drinking 'the black drink,' says Gen. Dale, is this: When they are
all seated around one of them takes the gourd, (kept for that purpose)
holds it over the pot, pours into it the liquid and continues pouring
in until it foams and runs over. He then takes the gourd to the
Head Chief and begins making a long note, drawing out his breath
longer than one would suppose he could; he then draws his breath a
second time, giving another long note, but in a different key. He
then carries the gourd to the other chiefs, giving each of them a
grunt as he presents it. There is no fixed time for the latter to
drink by; the head chief drinks during the making of the two notes.
They drink a quart at a time as hot as they can bear it. Some 15
minutes afterwards they vomit the drink without any effort or
artificial means. The virtue of the drink is exhiliration and warmth
to the system." [29]

Bossu says:

"All the savages of the country of the Alabamas drink cassine;
it is the leaf of an extremely bushy shrub; it is not larger than a
black poplar (liard) but is serrated all around. They roast it as
we make coffee, and drink the infusion with many ceremonies. When
this diuretic drink is made, the young people go to offer it in gourds
open like cups, according to the quality and rank of the chiefs and the
warriors; that is to say to the Honored men, then to the other warriors,
according to their rank. They preserve the same order when they
offer the calumet for smoking; while you drink they shout with a
loud voice and lessen it gradually; when you have stopped drinking
they catch their breath and when you begin again they continue
the same shouting. This kind of orgy lasts sometimes for six hours
in the morning until two hours after noon. These savages are not

[28] Journal of David Taitt, in Mereness, Trav. in Am. Col., pp. 502-503.
[29] Claiborne, Miss., vol. i, p. 491.

otherwise inconvenienced by their drinking, to which they attribute much virtue. They throw it up without effort and without inconvenience. The women never drink of this beverage which is made only for warriors. It is in such assemblies into which they (the women) are never admitted that they relate all of their news and deliberate over their political business, concerning war or peace." [30]

Milfort is another French traveler who has left us a description of this ceremonial:

"When the savages assemble for any reason they are accustomed before undertaking any business, to begin by smoking their pipes, and drinking a liquor which they make from the leaf of a tree, very common among them, and which it is claimed is a wild tea tree. It much resembles that of China, except that the leaf is much smaller. This tree is green during the entire year; its leaf is gathered only when it is to be served. When the savages wish to make use of it they have it boiled like coffee. When they prepare this liquor to drink in their assembly this is how they treat it. They put a certain quantity of tea leaves into an earthen vessel which they place over the fire; when they are dried sufficiently, they put in water in proportion to the quantity of leaves, and boil the whole. When they decide that the infusion is strong enough, they pass it through a basket like a sifter, and leave it in great earthen vessels destined to receive it for cooling. When it is not warmer than the natural heat of milk, one of the old men who has charge of this ceremony has it put into gourds at the top of which is an opening about two inches in diameter. It is presented for drinking in these gourds, and for this purpose it is passed in succession to each one of the members of the assembly."

He adds that it was later vomited up in order to assure clear headedness on the part of the members of the assembly in taking up the business in hand, particularly to insure against the effects of spirituous liquors. [31]

It is not clear that this ceremony was gone through on all occasions when the black drink was taken, because in some towns and at certain times it is said to have been taken every morning. In particular it was prescribed for those men who were appointed to preserve the buildings of the Tukabahchee Square. They were not permitted to eat until after they had taken it. It at least preceded all important assemblies. Adair, in pursuance of his pet theory of an Israelitish origin for the American Indians, lays great stress upon the syllables uttered by the bearers of the black drink, and he supposes that they were the syllables of the name Jehovah. It so happens that although I can add little or nothing regarding the ceremony in general I obtained a short account of it from Jackson Lewis which

[30] Bossu, Nouv. Voy., vol. II, pp. 41-42.
[31] Milfort, Mém., pp. 195-199.

throws light upon just this point. He stated that formerly the black drink (àsi) was taken at the same time as the busk medicines, though it has now long been abandoned. But, while those who take the ordinary busk medicines go to the medicine pots to drink, the black drink was brought to the drinkers by four bearers. Each of these men would hand a pot of àsi to one who was to drink and when the latter placed it to his lips the bearer would utter a cry, which, as described to me, was something like this, "ā-a-a-a-a-a-a-a-a-a-a-a-a-a dī—i-i-i-i-i-i-i-i-i-i," both syllables being drawn out very long and gradually fading away. The drinker had to keep on imbibing the liquid until this cry came to an end. The cry was called the cry of the Yahola, a being described already, who with his companion Hayuya presided particularly over the square ground,[32] and it appears to have been uttered on other occasions, as for instance by the official who drew circles on the square ground just before the women's dance to indicate where the women were to stand. It is also said to have been applied to the cry used in calling a youth out when a new war name was to be conferred upon him. By some the medicine bearers were believed to be imitating the rapid fluttering of certain beetles or wasps, and the cries which they made were supposed to be in imitation of them, but this may have been merely an association by analogy. Questions of precedence were very carefully observed in the serving of àsi and were, I am informed, an occasion for frequent quarrels.

MINOR CEREMONIES CONNECTED WITH THE SQUARE GROUNDS

The communal grounds with their various appurtenances were, of course, laid out in a new place with great ceremony. I have already given all that I know regarding the ceremonies performed in putting up the tcokofa.[33] The planting of the ceremonial ball post also took place with certain peculiar observances.

Wiley Buckner, a leading man among the Okchai Indians, said that he had heard that the Alabama Indians before setting up a new post laid a scalp down, placed a stone over that and set the butt end of the post above. Woksi mi'ko, a Hilibi Indian, had heard that, when the Okchai were going to put up a new post, they went into the woods, selected a pine tree suitable for the purpose, and felled it so that it would come down on some logs without touching the ground. Then they cut all of the sap wood away, leaving only the heart of the tree. This done, a number of persons would go out to it, raise it, and carry it to the place where it was to be erected without letting it touch the ground. They would then bring a scalp taken from an

[32] See p 485.
[33] See pp. 177-181.

enemy, place it at the bottom of the hole prepared for the pole, and set the pole over it. While this operation was taking place the men engaged in it abstained from food—and probably went through some medicine ceremony—during seven days. Sanger Beaver, an old man of Tcatoksofka, the busk ground of which has long been given up, remembered seeing such a ceremony himself at a time when he was just old enough to take any notice of the customs of his people. He remembered that on one occasion, after they had cleared off the square ground and while they were still fasting, a great crowd of men went into the bottoms and cut down a very tall tree.[34] Without letting this fall to the ground they brought it to the busk ground and dug a hole for it. Then one of the henihas brought a human skull and deposited it at the bottom. They set the pole above this, and afterwards ran around it four times, shouting. Finally the man who had brought the skull climbed to the top of the pole and fixed there a wooden figure of a bird.

When beds were erected for a new ground those who had seats in each vied with one another to see which bed should be up first, and the party which won made great sport of the others as if they had won a ball game. The extra bed for the women and children was finished by all working together.

Big Jack, one of the leading Hilibi Indians, said that before establishing a new fire in the square ground after it had been moved they took some ashes from the old fire and buried them about a foot under ground in the place where the new fire was to be made. A doctor conjured these and repeated a formula over them as he put them in place. A small stone was also brought from the miko's bed in the old square ground and placed under the new one in the same manner. It was to show that the miko ought to be settled like a rock and a man of weight. The posts of the beds—which properly should be eight— particularly the front posts, had to be conjured and some hitci pàkpàgi put into each post hole. The same informant added that all foundations must be started with hitci pàkpàgi, which may therefore have been used under the ball post also. The removal of ashes from old to new fireplaces was confirmed by others and so was the use of hitci pàkpàgi under the posts, but I heard nothing further about the stone. Two of the leading Coweta Indians and a Tulsa Indian said that under their old fire in Alabama the Coweta had a "can" of medicine supposed to contain the dried residue of the first medicine ever used in the old country. It was about an arm's length under ground. When they emigrated to Oklahoma this medicine was dug up, carried along with the emigrants, and buried in the same way underneath the fire in the first busk ground on the Arkansas River. But when the square was again moved the medicine was not dug up, and it is supposed to be in the same place. These

[34] He called it a cedar, but there seems to be some doubt on this point.

men also affirmed that all Creek towns had such a "can" of medicine, but I am not certain of this. Perhaps they were thinking of the custom of removing ashes from the old fire. However, the Tulsa Indian to whom reference has been made asserted that there was such a custom, and that when the Coweta and Kasihta Indians separated they divided the contents of the medicine "can." The "can" at Coweta was declared to be about 14 inches long by 4 in diameter.

An Okmulgee Indian told me that when the old Lutcapoga busk ground was laid out the Creeks would not use animals to bring out the posts and other timbers but carried them 4 or 5 miles on their shoulders or by means of other sticks run under them.

The Great Annual Ceremony or Busk

The word "busk" is a traders' corruption of the native Creek poskita or boskita meaning "a fast." This term was of course applied to many different kinds of fasts, but to two above all, first the fast undergone by those desiring to become doctors or learned men, in the manner to be described presently,[35] and second the great annual ceremonial ushering in the Creek New Year.

Without doubt there was a long myth relating the origin of this observance and probably detailing how it was to be conducted. Probably there were several such myths. Indeed fragments are preserved in Chekilli's migration legend and in those recorded by Hawkins, Gatschet, and others,[35a] but the Creeks of the present day for the most part know only that it was established in the beginning of things for the benefit of the Indians and that its observance is thought to keep them and their families in good health throughout the ensuing year. A Kasihta informant said that when God made the earth he put in these medicines to be used for the good of the Indians and decreed that they must obey the instructions of the old people. A Coweta Indian also said that the busk customs were given by God when he made the world. Big Jack of Hilibi affirmed that Ibofánga (The-One-Above) gave the Indians the pasa and the miko hoyanĭdja to keep as long as time should last. Alindja, a Tukabahchee, maintained also that Ibofánga laid the foundation of the fire and gave the medicines to go with it. A Hilibi Indian said that the busk was given by God in earliest times for the good of the Indians, and it was said that all would be well so long as it was kept up. Jackson Lewis merely stated that the origin of the busk had "gone into the mist."

More specific was the information obtained by one of the Tulsa Indians from an old Alabama. This was to the effect that the busk medicines were sent down from God by two old gray-headed men.

---

[35] See pp. 617–620.　　　[35a] See pp. 33–68.

As soon as the old men had delivered them they disappeared, returning to the sky. According to Tál mutcási, the medicine maker of
Asilanabi and Lálogálga, seven selected men were putting the four
logs together to make a foundation, and, as they were making the
foundation, "there was a fire built" and it was said of the four
main sticks: "They shall be the white path. There shall be peace
and harmony." At this time were established the laws by which
the people were to be ruled. They were also given the medicine
roots and were told "This shall be your medicine. This shall be
respected and appreciated as long as time lasts."

Still another story is from Sanger Beaver, a Tcatoksofka Indian.
He had heard that in ancient times the people were continually
fighting, scalping, and killing, were without law, and went about
nearly naked, clothed only in the skin breechclout. A certain man
among them meditated much on this troublesome way of living.
He fasted and thought for a long time, and finally he declared that
he had received "the white day" (ni'ta hátki). This had been given
to man through him by Ibofánga along with the miko hoyanídja,
the pasa, the sawátcka, and the ási, and songs for each medicine.
These were, to quote the language of this anonymous person, "for
the building up of our future generations, to make grow up the
women and the children." Having said this he started the fire of
the confederacy by using four sticks of wood, and the other Indian
tribes came there and obtained their fires from the one kindled by
that old Indian. For this reason the Creeks claimed to be the
originators of all of the national fires of the various Indian nations.
Beaver added the important information that most of this story is
contained in a kind of song that had been handed down from the
old Indian that received the "white day." There is, of course, very
much more to the story, but he did not know the rest. From such
an origin grew the customs and practices of the busk, and it is said
that the tribe was instructed that so long as it adhered to the use
of these medicines, customs, etc., it would grow strong, but if at any
time they became lax in attending to them they would grow weak
and perish. The busk and the stomp dances which preceded it
were all for the sake of the tribal health.

Many of the Indians claim that the first busk fire was built in the
town of Tukabahchee and that all of the other towns derived their
fire from that source, but I have shown elsewhere that this is a later
explanation. It is admitted, nevertheless, by nearly all of the other
Upper Creek towns. By some, all of their laws and regulations are
traced to the Ispokogis and presumably the busk fires also. It is
also said that when the Shawnee came east into the country of the
Creeks they found that the stomp ground and the busk were not
quite "right" and they remodeled them. Then they returned to

their home in the west and one town followed them. This may indicate nothing more than the high regard in which the Shawnee were held. Certain innovations in the busk procedure may have been due to them, but to prove it we must wait for a study of Shawnee ceremonials.

The story of Sanger Beaver probably represents very well the psychological attitude of the Indians toward their great ceremonial and epitomizes their opinion of its place in their lives even though it may not have the slightest basis in fact. The busk with its fire, its medicines, and its ceremonial was a great unifying element between the several members of the Creek confederacy, all the tribes which united with it either adopting such a ceremonial or altering their own to agree with it. And further than that it was a special unifying institution within each town, bringing all together for a definite purpose in which the good of each and the good of all were bound up. All transgressions, except some forms of murder, were then forgiven, all disturbances adjusted, and thus the unity and peace of the state reestablished. As with so many reputed founders of civilized states in the Old World, and as in the case of Hiawatha among the Iroquois, a primeval age of barbarism and warfare is put an end to by a lawgiver acting as the medium of supernatural agents, or possessing great supernatural power. The object of his labors is law, order, and peace. Thus the busk is supposed to be a great peace ceremonial, "the white day," the square ground is considered "the yard of peace," white feathers are used there, and its white smoke is intended to reach the sky. The White clans and Tcilokis were to play peaceably in the ball game and the side which won was to take both bunches of feathers. When a council of any kind was held, pipes were lighted and smoked, and the smoke ascending from them was called "the white smoke." As Swan tells us, the native name of the sacred medicine called "black drink" by the whites is really "the white drink." It is now claimed that the four foundation sticks of the fire depict the junction lines of "the white treaty" with the United States Government, and an old Tukabahchee Creek said that the White people promised to be on the north end of the north back stick of the busk fire. This interpretation, however, has evidently superseded an earlier one in which the Creek confederacy as represented by its four leading towns, Coweta, Kasihta, Tukabahchee, and Abihka, was symbolized by the fire sticks. The fact that the beds of the miko and henihas are often spoken of as white and were usually occupied by White clans also shows the dominance of the idea of peace in the square ground and particularly the busk ceremonial held there. It is to be added that at the time of this ceremonial everyone must speak in a low, gentle tone of voice, if children begin to cry, they must be quieted at once without disturbance, and a general air of harmony must be preserved.

If it may be relied upon as a common belief the following information obtained by Doctor Speck from Laslie Cloud, medicine maker of the Tuskegee, is very valuable:

"Upon the same occasion (the busk) the clan totems and other animal spirits are worshiped and propitiated by numerous dances each with its own song and gestures. These address prayer and express gratitude to the propitious ones and correspondingly placation to those that are believed to be nocuous. To take an example, the *stikini*, 'little screech owl,'[35b] is an unfavorable spirit of the dead, causing death or announcing death to the one who hears it. So the *Stikino-bánga*, 'Little-screech-owl dance,' is functionally a prayer to the screech owl for immunity from its visits. These dances are performed publicly on the square ground and all spectators may take part freely. In other cases dances are directed, as acts of worship by emulation, to the spirits of animals whose flesh is food. The emulation is believed to affect the spirits of the dead animals in their reincarnation upon the earth. So with the fish dance, the buffalo dance, and others."[36]

Unfortunately I have been entirely unable to substantiate this even at the mouths of very intelligent old people and consequently do not know whether it was the personal understanding of Laslie Cloud or represented a former widely extended belief. But since the busk was a very sacred ceremonial a symbolic meaning was likely to be extended over every feature connected with it.

But we must not lose sight of the fact that the "peace" of the busk was a peace with limitations. It included the town busking, it included in a lesser degree the other Creek towns of the same fire, and in a lesser degree still the towns of the other fire, the contests with which were merely through ball games, but here it stopped and, just as peace and ball games were institutional up to that point, so was war institutional beyond that point. War was by no means excluded from consideration in the square ground and the busk, or even temporarily suppressed. The warriors had their distinctive beds where they were ranged in grades, advancement in the seatings, and along with it new names, was granted for achievements in almost all cases obtained in war, the warriors had their definite part in the ceremonies, and the atásá, the war symbol, was given to the youth who was thus renamed, carried by the women who led the women's dance, and indicated by short posts or by markings upon the tall posts in the front of the beds of the chief himself.[37] Atásá posts

---

[35b] This is really the horned owl.

[36] Speck in Mem. Am. Anth. Asso., vol. II, pt. 2, pp. 134–135.

[37] It is now denied that there is any ceremonial meaning to the atásá sticks carried by the women in the women's dance or to the feathers which the young men like to stick in their hats, but both are undoubtedly descended from significant usages.

are shown in Figure 5 of the preceding paper, from an early French sketch.[38]   As in the reform movement of Hiawatha among the Iroquois and similar reforms in other parts of the world, that perception of the injurious effects of war with which the confederacy started was not carried on progressively toward its legitimate conclusion, the absolute extinction of warfare, but halted part way.   In the relative benefits which the new union conferred by introducing local peace were lost to sight the very much greater benefits which would have been conferred by carrying out the project to its only logical end. The local well being and warlike effectiveness of a certain group of tribes was very much advanced as compared with that of many of their neighbors, and with this they remained content.

The busk was in reality the fourth of a series of ceremonials, the first three of which are called "stomp dances" and included only a minimum of ceremony, being in a way preparatory to the great busk proper.   It is likely that in ancient times these were of more importance and perhaps deserved the name of busk also.   The time of these ceremonies was formerly fixed by the period of the new moon and therefore varied somewhat.   The first stomp dance was usually in April, but sometimes probably in May, while the busk proper was usually in July but with some towns as late as August.   In ancient times the date of the busk was supposed to be governed by the first ripening of the large or flour corn,[39] and this will account for the fact that among the Florida Seminole it is said to occur as early as June.[40]

The Koasati observed one of the three first stomp dances with more than ordinary care.   It was the one held in May and was when the mulberries were ripe.   It will be remembered that Adair says of the Koasati that "they annually sanctify the mulberries by a public oblation,"[41] and I was told as much by David Cummings, probably the only Creek living in 1912 who could remember about the old busk ground of the main body of Koasati, known as Koasati No. 1.   He said that they busked in May when the mulberries were ripe and again when the roasting ears were ripe.   Stiggins states that the Koasati celebrated the coming of the new crop of beans in addition to the coming of the new corn, and this was probably identical with the mulberry feast.[41a]

The following feast mentioned by Adair was perhaps at the time of one of these stomp dances—at least it was at the same time of the year—although there are features reminding one of the "old peoples' dance" which the Creeks held in October.   Adair says of this feast:

[38] Journ. Société des Amér. de Paris, 1922.
[39] Adair says it was anciently fixed by "the beginning of the first new moon in which their corn became full eared," but later by the time of harvest. (Hist. Am. Inds., p. 99.)
[40] See MacCauley, Fifth Ann. Rept. Bur. Ethn.
[41] Adair, Hist. Am. Inds., p. 267.
[41a] See p. 568.

"Every spring season, one town or more of the Mississippi Flor-
idians, keep a great solemn feast of love, to renew their old friendship.
They call this annual feast, Hottuk Aimpa, Heettla, Tanaa [háták ai-
impa, hila, tánaa], 'the people eat, dance, and walk as twined together.' [42]   The short name of their yearly feast of love, is Hottuk
Impanaa, 'eating by a strong religious, or social principle.' [43]

"They assemble three nights previous to their annual feast of
love; on the fourth night they eat together. During the intermediate
space, the young men and women dance in circles from evening
till morning. The men masque their faces with large pieces of gourds
of different shapes and hieroglyphic paintings. Some of them fix a
pair of young buffalo horns to their head; others the tail, behind.
When the dance and their time is expired, the men turn out a hunting, and bring in a sufficient quantity of venison, for the feast of renewing their love, and confirming their friendship with each other.
The women dress it, and bring the best they have along with it;
which a few springs past, was only a variety of Esau's small red acorn
pottage, as their crops had failed. When they have eaten together,
they fix in the ground a large pole with a bush tied at the top, over
which they throw a ball. Till the corn is in, they meet there almost
every day, and play for venison and cakes, the men against the
women; which the old people say they have observed for time out
of mind." [44]

The Creek year was divided, as explained elsewhere, into two
seasons of six months each and the busk in July or August marked
the beginning of the new year, from which they counted at least
every event of a sacred nature.[45] Another division at right angles to
this might, however, be made, into a ceremonial and nonceremonial
season, the former from April to about October, the latter including
the balance of the year. It is by no means certain that there were
no regular public ceremonies during the strictly winter months, but
no proof of their existence survives. On the other hand there is a
very coherent account of the summer ceremonies and feasts, showing
them to have extended in an almost unbroken series from comparatively early in the spring until late in the fall. I have a fairly clear
outline of this from Mr. Ellis Childers, the last chief of the Chiaha
before they gave up their busk ground, and a man of former prom-
inence in the affairs of the Creek Nation.

"When the new moon at the end of April or beginning of May
approaches the medicine man (hilis-haya) tells the miko to call
his people.[46] He also tells the miko in what phase of the moon to

---

[42] Tána means to knit, weave, or plait.
[43] There seems to be no especial religious connotation in these words.
[44] Adair, Hist. Am. Inds., pp. 113–114. Cf. pp. 525–526, 555–556; 404 in preceding paper.
[45] Ibid., pp. 76–77.
[46] Hawkins says that the date of the Kasihta busk was fixed by the miko and his counselors.

send out. Immediately the miko sends a ta'pala or 'messenger' through the town to notify everyone to meet at the square-ground that night. They gradually assemble during the day. After all is ready they generally dance the obanga hadjo until midnight, when the medicine-maker orders the miko to prepare for the next day. The miko then directs certain men to dig the medicine plants. That night the men sleep on the square ground, and next morning each medicine hunter goes to get the medicine he is to provide. The principal of these is the miko hoyanidja. Others are the pasa, cedar, and a plant called hitū'tàbi, 'ice weed,' about which ice accumulates on frosty mornings. Those medicines which consisted of the boughs of trees were taken from the east side. On their return these men lay each of the medicines in a certain designated place. Then officers appointed called 'medicine mixers' place all of the medicines except the pasa in one pot. All go into this at the same time except the miko hoyanidja and cedar. Formerly there were four pots of medicine which were used at as many different times during the night; in later times only two pots were used.

"It should be mentioned that cedar twigs must be tied to the middle post of each bed in front, and sometimes such twigs are tied on the corner posts also.

"The miko hoyanidja is tied into four bunches, a certain amount going into each. This is generally done by the diggers. The medicine mixers now take one bunch of miko hoyanidja, wash it, beat the bark off, and put all into the pot containing the mixture. These men have entire charge of the handling of the medicine pots throughout. In the meantime two messengers of the chief called ta'pala secure buckets and place them in front of those persons sitting on the beds who are to bring water. They must bring this from a running stream, and some of it is then added to the medicine in the pots. The medicine being now ready the medicine man takes a long cane and blows into it, usually four times, generally chanting as he does so. Then the chief usually stands up in his place, and one of the medicine mixers takes a bucket of medicine and a cedar bush. He dips the bush into the medicine and sprinkles a little over each bed and over the entire square ground. One bucket of medicine is set apart, and the medicine maker blows into this in the same way as before. Afterward, one of the medicine mixers goes through the same sprinkling process again, first calling up and sprinkling all those who have dug graves or handled dead bodies in any manner. Then each medicine mixer seizes a bucket, and they carry the medicine to each person present. About one or two quarts is given to each, and for this purpose each person is supposed to bring a cup; if he does not, a cup is supplied.

"After all have taken the medicine and vomited they wait a certain time and then the second bunch of miko hoyanidja is mixed in, the pot being refilled with water. The medicine is then passed around again, and the same process is gone through four times in all during the day, once for each bunch of miko hoyanīdja. Each time the medicine maker blows into the pot before it is distributed. The pasa is used but once and is the last drink of the day. It is slightly warmed over a little fire. Generally it is not mixed until after the medicine has been taken for the third time. Roots of the wormseed [46a] (wīlana) are dug and many of them placed on a near-by bench. After the last drink they march out to the creek to bathe, and on the way each takes a few wormseed roots, chews and swallows a little, and rubs his head thoroughly with them, after which he dives into the creek four times. This completes the ceremonies for the day.

"During the intervals between the taking of the medicine the business of the town is attended to. In cases of misunderstandings and quarrels between persons or families the parties are questioned, either by the chief or by those whom he selects, generally persons from the henihas' bench, who finally determine which way the dispute should be settled. When the decision is agreed upon, the parties are called up and informed, and almost invariably they abide by this judgment.

"After they have returned from bathing the participants are allowed to eat, and in the evening after dark they are summoned to the square. A dance then begins in the ball ground to the southeast of the square ground, and they start with a song in which certain things are done at intervals in keeping with the words. Finally, at a particular, understood place, they march in around the fire in the square ground. A dance leader is now selected by the chief's messengers (ta'palas). Dances now follow each other, one after the other, all night, but at intervals the chief makes speeches, and he also invites good speakers who happen to be present to address the people. In that way good advice is given regarding the proper conduct of the rising generation and the proper way of living. It is the chief's duty to inform the people in this way of any occurrence which concerns his town. He imparts the messages which he has received from other towns, and which come through him, to his people. This assembly is thus an aid to government. Next morning the meeting breaks up and the people go home.

"At the next new moon the same performance is gone through. On the new moon after that a third meeting is held. On the morning of the day when this meeting opens all of the male members of the town are requested to be present in the square and the chief and a chosen number from each bed decide upon the date for the annual

---

[46a] Usually but erroneously called "Jerusalem oak." I am indebted to Mr. Paul C. Standley, of the U. S. National Museum, for the correction.

busk. Then a switch cane is split up into pieces about the size of a match, and bunches are made of these, each bunch containing as many sticks as there are days to the time of the great busk. Each is tied up with a buckskin string. One of these bundles is tied immediately over the chief's seat in the square. Each of the others is sent to one of the friendly towns—that is, those of the same fire clan—as an invitation to share with them in the annual busk. It is immediately delivered to the town chief of that town by the ta'palas appointed by the town chief.

"The fourth day before the date of the busk is known as 'camping day'; on this all must be encamped about the square ground. The next day is known as 'visitors' day' when all visitors are looked after and provided with camping quarters. The third day is known as 'the feast day,' on which food is kept prepared all day, so that one can help himself whenever he wants to. The day is generally passed in playing ball, either the men's game being played or the one-pole game between men and women. The fourth day is the 'busk day' in which medicine is taken. Medicine is gathered, mixed, and taken as already described for the stomp-dance. Up to the time of this busk the inhabitants of the town have been forbidden to eat certain vegetable productions, the principal of which is green corn, and from this fact is derived the term 'green corn dance.' In case one has eaten green corn before this time, medicine is administered to him before the general medicine taking, and he is also scratched on the muscles of the arms and legs, four scratches being made with a one-pointed needle or one scratch with a four-pointed one. The scratches made were pretty deep. In olden times the snout of a garfish was employed exclusively.

"On the afternoon of 'visitors' day' friendly relations are shown by an exchange of tobacco. The people of the town giving the busk are seated on their beds, and the visitors, marching in, offer a piece of tobacco to each, beginning with the chief, saying at the same time 'Partake of this with me.' After they have taken it each of the town people, beginning with the chief, offers the leader of the visitors a piece of tobacco in his turn. This exchange has superseded the custom of smoking together, when a large pipe was filled with tobacco and passed from hand to hand. The order observed was probably N E S W, the chief sending around to the beds successively in this direction.[47] The chief of the visitors then took a pipe around in turn, beginning at the west bed where was the chief. All orders were given by the town chief to a ta'pala (who was not necessarily a heniha) and by him to the people. This pipe, therefore, was first lighted by the chief and by him given to the ta'pala to be carried along.

---

[47] The correctness of this is doubted.

"On the morning of the 'busk day,' after breakfast and before the medicine has been prepared, the visitors return home. First, however, they march up in a line and pass the southeast corner; as they do so they wave their right hands in unison toward the square so as to take it all in and say apokatcges ayīpaläs ('While you abide I will return'), a friendly expression. In reply the people of the town respond hō ('Yes,' 'All right,' or 'Very well').

"To make the fire, four green sticks are cut from tree limbs extending toward the east. These are known as 'the back logs' (tăkhudji). To renew the fire they use the term to'hsoloti', 'to shove them in together.' Four roasting-ears are placed across the back sticks, as in Figure 108. Then kindling, hay, or other dry stuff is placed on top and ignited by rubbing two dry sticks lengthwise [?] over it. Fire can be started very quickly in this way. All the fires in the camps have meanwhile been put out, and this new fire is taken to them. It is used for the first time in cooking the first meal after the men break their fast. All disputes have now been settled by the henīhas and a new life begins.

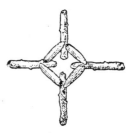

FIG. 108. — Arrangement of ears of corn on the fire sticks at the Chiaha busk

"After invitation sticks have been sent, anyone who fails to appear at the busk is considered disobedient to the chief, and on the morning when the busk breaks up the chief calls together the leaders of each bed and they make a list of all those who have failed to attend. Then a number of messengers (ta'pala) are sent to these individuals to collect a fine which is said to have amounted to $2.50 in cash. It is customary to send to each man someone of the clan to which he himself belongs. When the ta'pala arrives he seizes any animal the man may have that is eatable, kills it, and brings it back to the square. It has been agreed upon on what day the fines shall be brought to the square, and then a second feast is called to eat up these things.

"This feast initiates a series of games between the women and men, wherein a wager is made—generally between a man and his 'sister-in-law,' i. e., a woman who has married into his clan. The man wagers part of a deer, while the woman puts up a pot of blue dumplings, or some sofki, or both. This game is played once a week for three weeks, and after the third a day is set for the hunters to go out. A day for finishing the fourth game is also agreed upon between the parties who made the wager. At that time the deer or other game is brought to the square ground and delivered to the woman who made the wager, she being encamped there with other women to assist her. Among the things that they feast upon that day is a great pot of soup, and the feast is therefore called 'the soup-drinking feast.' This wager having been concluded another pair lays a wager in the same manner and the same games and feasts are repeated. The night of each of these feasts they generally dance all night, and commonly they have one every month. The town chief is present if possible, and if anything should keep him away, the second chief takes his place. This series of feasts generally extends through the warm weather until it begins to get cool, the latter part of September or the first part of October, and the season is closed by what they call 'the last dances.' One of these is known as 'the old men's dance,' and another is the 'wolf dance.' The first has been discontinued for a number of years, especially by the Chiaha, because all of those who were able to lead it have died. I saw only one and that when I was a boy. I can not give details regarding the conduct of it, but it is different from anything else I ever saw or heard of. As nearly as I can remember the men went off and dressed in masks, some representing bear, some wolves, panthers, or even cattle, bulls, etc., or perhaps a band of Indians of some foreign tribe. Others dressed in still other ways, but all appeared as very old people. They seemed to represent dramatically an event in hunting, an attack by some dangerous animal, and their conquest over it by means of their skill and experience as old men. A number of ceremonies took place in connection with this dance; women also took part. This dance was held in all of the Creek towns.[48]

"To dance the Wolf Dance the men rise very early on a day that has been previously fixed upon and meet at the square, each riding his best pony. The men who take part in this dance are principally the young men of the town. They then proceed to the nearest house, generally at full speed, yelling, whooping, and singing. On reaching the house, all dismount and they dance around it, their leader singing a song, the rest whooping and yelling in discord to represent the howling of wolves. Then the inmates set out some food, and each of the dancers rushes up and snatches a little of it and runs off with it. Having eaten this they proceed to the next house and the same thing is repeated. So they visit all of the houses in the neighborhood. Afterward they return home, but that afternoon all meet at the square and at night they have the dance. The dances that night, especially those begun after midnight, are different from the regular stomp dances. Among these are the horse dance, the duck dance, the chicken dance, the catfish dance, a dance called a 'double dance' in which there are two leaders, etc. Next morning just as the sun rises they close the season by dancing the 'drunken man's dance.' Meanwhile the chief is generally present to communicate the news, and the henihas are always about to compose differences."

---

[48] For another description see p. 534.

CREEK RELIGION AND MEDICINE

This sequence is no longer preserved in anything like its ancient completeness, those feasts that follow the busk especially having dropped out of use, but the busk itself still (1912) holds on in about eleven towns not counting the Yuchi and in six Seminole towns. In some of these, for instance the Tukabahchee, the three stomp dances are kept up in some form, and in fact my most complete account of the three stomp dances and the busk is from Zachariah Cook, a former miko of Tukabahchee town. This is as follows:

"At the end of the busk the chief says to his people 'Go home and do the best you can, and next year when the moon is about at such and such a place I will send you the "broken days." When the time approaches, which is near the time of the new moon in April, he sends a bunch of seven little sticks to the head man in each neighborhood who throws one stick away each day, and leaves home so as to get to the square ground on the night of the seventh day. On the eighth they fast all day and tásikayas, under the supervision of the imałas, work for the hilis-haya (medicine maker), each getting four shoulder loads of wood. After that they are told to prepare for the all night dance. A man called itci yahola dances the war dance (paihka obánga, "whooping dance") with a scalp and a toma- hawk. They give him a fawn skin and a ribbon and he is the leader in the women's dance. Owing to this fact the women plant his field for him—at least the two leaders of the women called tcukoleidji do so and sometimes the others help.[48a] The same day they procure new brooms if any are needed. Then all are told to go and rest and abstain from eating. They take that time for the performance of necessary duties such as watering horses. Early that same morning four persons, two isti-àtcagagi-sûlgas and two henihas, are sent to dig miko hoyanīdja. The tconoh hola'ta is called up and sent with one of the henihas to get the cedar and other ingredients of the warm medicine. The medicine is placed at the north end of the west bed. Two youths are then called up to fix the medicine. They go for water, and after they have brought it put hitci pàkpàgi in each pot as a foundation for the 'warm bath.' The rest of the ten medicines are piled upon this, and the whole is called adiloga or atiloga. Then they get rocks, pound up the miko hoyanīdja and put it into another vessel side of the first. After that they get cánes and straighten them and tell the hilis-haya that all is ready. They provide a deerskin for him to sit on and another for a footstool.

"The hilis-haya then blows into the medicines, and an old heniha sitting close to him summons another, and they remove the pots, placing the atiloga on the north side by the fire and the miko hoyanīdja just west of it. Then the old henīha who was sitting by the hilis-haya gets one gourdful of each medicine and gives it to

_____

48a At Tukabahchee and Kealedji this field was close to the northwestern edge of the square ground.

the miko and his henîha who lay it in the bed right back of them. The miko then summons the two youths who mixed the medicine and he and his henîha hand the gourds to them, after which they go round inside close to the beds, keeping the fire on the left, the isti-àtcagàgi-sûlga in the lead, and they sprinkle the medicines toward the beds with their hands. This is to prevent the spirits of the dead from interfering. These gourds are then returned to the bed back of the miko. This circuit is performed four times during the night, the youths being called up each time for that purpose. Through his henîha the miko then summons the speaker who rises and shouts as loudly as he can for all the men to come inside of the grounds. All the women remain outside. Having assembled, the men are notified that they must fast that day, but that all who had handled the dead are to wait and take their medicine afterward. Then the medicine is taken in the following order: miko, speaker (yatika), miko's henîha, the other mikos, the two youths who sprinkled medicine, the Wind clan, tàstànàgàlgi, imalàlgi, isti-àtcagagi-sûlga, Bird clan, and the other clans down to the Panther and the Potato which is usually last. They take first the warm medicine and then the cold, and go afterward to vomit them out. Now the miko summons two ta'palas, a Raccoon and a Wind usually, though if necessary some other clan is substituted for the Raccoon, to manage the dance, and he tells them to choose a dance leader to keep the dance going. This is done while the drinking is still going on so that by the time it is over the miko can call out 'There is a dance leader over yonder.' When this leader starts all get out and help him, and after they have danced the common, or 'stomp' dance (sătkita obànga) four times the women come in with rattles on their ankles and prepare to dance. When they get a little tired of the common dances they may take up special dances such as the gar dance, buffalo dance, quail dance, duck dance, etc. The hînàtà dance is a very pretty one and so are the quail and horse dances. If they can get a capable singer who knows them they may dance these special dances all night; otherwise they keep on with the common dance. Finally a time is set for the second 'stomp' dance which proceeds in the same manner. The third dance is a big dance.

"At that dance a council is held by the isti-àtcagàgi-sûlga as to whether they will remodel their square ground, and if they decide to do so they set a time in the fall, perhaps in September, for carrying on this work. If the hot house is to be fixed up a time is also set in September. The same men are called in to arrange for the busk. They go over the entire program, one saying 'I will do this,' another 'I will do that,' and so on. Then they say 'We will meet ten days from tomorrow.' When they do meet they say 'We will meet in five days,' but they count in the day on which they make the arrangement and also the day of meeting at the end, therefore there are only three whole days between. At that meeting they say 'We will meet in three days,' but one day intervening; and then they say 'We will meet in two days,' meaning the next. Finally they say 'We will meet in one day,' but they mean the very same day, so they simply go back home and then return, clear the ground off, and prepare the 'broken days,' of little canes, seven to the bundle, a bundle for each neighborhood. The messenger who delivers these pulls one stick out and throws it away, and afterward the head man at that place does the same each day until the time has arrived. When this distribution of sticks is made, they send a bundle to every fire of the same fire clan. The Atasi used to come down and busk with the Tukabahchee until the last dance, the women's dance, when they took some of the medicine which had been prepared for them and carried it back to their own women, who finished the dance. The Kēaledji simply sent two men to Tukabahchee for the new fire, which they carried home in a pot, putting new fuel in this from time to time until they got back. The Łapłako used to do like the Atasi, but later they got a hilis-haya of their own and tried to have their own ceremonial, but they soon gave it up. The Łiwahali also brought their fire from Tukabahchee. Hilibi and Eufaula acted more or less together and had their own fires. This was in late times.

"The day of the last meeting when the ground was cleared the leaders of the women, the tcukolaidji, came to the ground and sat on a small bench in a cleared space in the southwest corner. They helped some in clearing the yard except their own space which they did not touch.

"On the fifth day of the seven all the people are supposed to be at the busk ground. On the night of the fifth the miko appoints a man of the Deer clan, which is a 'choice clan,' as an 'orderly' (lā'ta mi'kàgi) to manage the women's dance. He brings him in and puts him next to the post at the south end of the center section of the Chiefs' bed. The same night the miko empowers two youths to call in the small boys, who come into the square and have a jolly dance in which women and girls also join. While this is going on the 'orderly' calls up the itci yahola and a henīha. A cane a yard long is given to each and they are sent to see how the preparations of the women for the dance next day are advanced and whether leaders have been selected, so that everything will be ready that night. After that four singers have to be called up, the ones who are to sing for the women next day. These singers have a waiter (saogadjilaia) who prepares the gourds, wraps their handles with hickory bark, etc., and places them in the back part of the youths' bed so that they may be ready in the morning. The 'orderly' then calls up a speaker and instructs him what he is to do and after that a drummer. By this time it is 10 or 11 o'clock at night and the women and young people go home, while the men stay on the busk ground, inside of the beds or around the ceremonial post, and sleep there.

"Very early on the following morning the 'orderly' prepares a little pot of miko hoyanïdja and places it in a little entrance between the center posts at the back of the Chiefs' bed. A little hitci pákpági is put into it first as a 'foundation,' the miko hoyanïdja and water are added, and finally the hilis-haya blows into it. Then the 'orderly' summons the itci yahola and henïha who had gone out before, gives each a little piece of tobacco, and tells them to go and ask the women to hasten. They go around four times to call them. If they still delay, these officials stand upon a little mound belonging to the women at the southwestern angle and shout to hurry them. The leaders of the women and the male officials fast. The women are dressing during this time, and they drift in to the rallying place until 10 or 11 o'clock. The man who prepared the gourd rattles has to move them (the rattles) to the end of the Panther bed. One of the henïhas is also sent to get the small pot of miko hoyanïdja and set it down in the little yard at the southwest corner, where the women take it and put it on their turtle-shell rattles and other paraphernalia. There are three leaders for the women, but there could be a fourth and probably that is the proper number. The leaders are a Raccoon, a Wind, a Panther (and a Bird). When they are ready the first woman, carrying her rattle, goes a short distance and stops; then woman number two follows her example and the same with woman number three who leads the crowd. Meanwhile, the miko has been calling the same two men repeatedly, giving them tobacco and sending them to hurry things up. The gourd rattles are put overhead in the Panthers' bed in front, then moved to a position close to the corner post, and again to the center of the Panthers' bed where the singers can reach them.[49] The speaker and singers also have to be ordered up. Meanwhile the women have to be drilled and prepared, and the itci yahola is called over to the Chiefs' bed to receive a deer skin and ribbons. Four dog-whippers are appointed for the corners of the square. Before the women come in the speaker gives orders to the drummer, who is out on the tádjo, a mound of earth back of the warriors' cabin, to beat his drum and at the fourth beat the men have to be in their places. A little basket is set down in front of the speaker, and he tells the women to bring small pieces of tobacco and throw them into it. Then he gives them a lecture, advising them to be silent, respectful, not too vulgar, etc. The Tcunuk hola'ta is called over, receives a paddle-shaped stick, and, following instructions, makes a circular mark on the ground in front of the east end of the Panthers' bed,

---

[49] Here the singers sit in the Panthers' bed; at Hilibi they sit on the end of the Raccoons' bed.

and a large circle around the fire. The former is the place where the leading woman is to stand and the large circle indicates where the rest are to range themselves. The speaker now calls the itci yahola who remains standing facing the north until he has been called twice. A fawn skin and ribbon are behind the miko and he hands them to the speaker who hands them in turn to the itci yahola standing to receive them. Holding these he goes through the circle of women and around some bushes which are set up in a circle about the fire, calling the yahola cry as he goes and holding his breath all the way around. When he gets back he says 'yux yu' as a mark of respect to the chief and then takes his seat. His henīha follows and takes his seat. The women dance two rounds, go out and rest, and then their leaders go out and bring them in for two more rounds.

"The miko next gets an īmala łáko and an īmala łábotski. In the first or second verse of a song, at least at a certain place in it, these īmalas run out and shout to the warriors 'Go and get the tea brush (ási sábonga)' meaning the brush with which to kindle the fire. All of the warriors then go for it. Now the henīha is told to call the fus isá 'to go and get the hickory bark,' meaning the punk with which the fire is started. Another henīha accompanies him, and they go out at the third or fourth verse (or song). Next four men are called up to get the four back sticks. They are instructed to secure sticks with the tops already broken off and such as they themselves can break off to a length of about four feet. These are placed at the end of the bed of the henihálgi. Six or eight youths are sent for the pasa and the same youths are sent again for the miko hoyanīdja. The dance is now over and they retire for that day. The people who remain have a ball game after dinner and a big time generally, and that night they have a jolly dance and afterward all retire, the men sleeping inside of the busk ground. The same night a man is selected to be captain over the young men and keep watch of them. The miko summons him next morning and tells him to assemble the youths and move the ashes of the old fires. From ten to fifty youths then set to work and soon have the ashes removed. Then the miko directs the leader to have them bring a lot of sand, which they move on boards, in their hands, or in any other way, and spread over the fireplace, covering a circle perhaps five feet in diameter. Then they are sent after more sand which they take out and spread back of the henihas' bed, on the site of the old hot house. If a little is left over it is put in front of the hilis-haya's place for the copper shields to rest upon. (From this point on the ceremony has now been modified. The older form which continues from here will be found on pp. 564–568.)

"Now the fire maker (tōtki dīdja) gets some blossoms of hitci pàkpàgi. The night before the miko has called eight or more isti àtcagàgi in person saying 'So-and-so, you must wake up in the morning early,' to each in turn. These men may call in some young fellows to help, and early in the morning they spread out a deer skin, lay down punk, and light a fire with flint and steel. In more ancient times they made a fire by rubbing two sticks together. The deer skin is on the seat on the north (or rather northwest) end of the Henīhas' bed. After the fire has been fed with a little bark most of it is removed from the skin, and what is left is used to kindle a little fire near the same end of this bed. Meantime the hilis-haya has made a cross-mark in the center of the square, the ends pointing toward the entrances between the cabins, and at the end of each and at the center he sets a piece of hitci pàkpàgi. The henīha is right behind him with four pieces of bark on which is fire and he places these in the center of the marks. The hilis-haya now goes and gets one of the four back sticks, conjures it, and sticks a little hitci pàkpàgi in the outer end of each. Then he lays it down pointing toward the west (or southwest) bed, just south of the line extending toward the west entrance. He then gets another stick, does the same with it, and places it toward the south (or southeast) bed. He does the same with the other two sticks, proceeding round the fire contra-clockwise. When all are in place he brushes one hand over the other with an outward sweep as a sign that the job is finished. Next lines are drawn, hitci pàkpàgi put in, and fire started on the site of the hot house, but no sticks are laid there. Finally the firemaker's henīha builds the small extra fire above mentioned at the end of the Henīhas' bed. A little pot of wormseed is now prepared in front of the Henīhas' bed, the hilis-haya blows into it, and moves it out to the third fire at the west end of the Warriors' bed.[50] It is placed near the fire there. The Wind clan, the henīhas, sat at the north end of the west or Chiefs' cabin, in what is ordinarily called the Chiefs' bed. This part of the cabin is called the Henīhas' bed.

"Eight roasting ears provided in advance are placed on the north end of the Henīhas' bed by the post. The husks of four are stripped back and tied together and they are hung overhead between the beds of the henihàlgi and mikàlgi. The oldest henīha brings the other four ears to the place where the medicine was prepared. The miko then gives the hilis-haya some hitci pàkpàgi, and the hilis-haya takes an ear of corn, blows on a blossom of hitci pàkpàgi and sticks it into one end of the ear. He lays this ear side of the back stick pointing to the west (toward the Chiefs' bed). He goes around the fire and comes back to the place from which he started. Then he

<hr/>

[50] Or "the north end of the Henīhas' bed"; my notes give it both ways. It is in the same entrance way in either case.

treats the ear for the south stick and the ones for the east and north sticks successively in the same manner. Finally he rubs one hand over the other to show that the work is completed.

"Now two ímalas are called who go out and notify the different camps to come and get the new fire. While they are doing this the medicine is being made. The captain of the youths is told to get them and go after the medicines. The oldest heníha already referred to as sitting by the post puts down a pounding-block with a deer skin over it for the hilis-haya to sit upon. It is placed right back of the medicine pots. The old heníha and a young boy of the heníhas now bring two pots for the medicine. They also bring up all of the pasa and all of the miko hoyanídja, but they select out of this for the hilis-haya four pasa plants and four sticks of miko hoyanídja. The hilis-haya now goes to the block covered with the deer skin and sits upon it. He lays a rock in front of him and uses another as a mallet. Then he takes one plant of pasa first, blows upon it, repeating some formula meanwhile, gives it one blow to break the roots off, and puts these into the pot. He does the same thing to the rest of the pasa and to the miko hoyanídja. The captain of the youths is now told to summon them and have them pound up the rest of the medicine and put it into the pots, which they do. The youths have already filled the pots with water.

"Now all retire and it is quiet for a space. On the morning of this day the little boys' busk is 'destroyed,' i. e., they cease to fast.

"Now the miko summons two waiters previously selected, one from the Raccoon clan and one from the Wind clan. He tells them to go out, fill two pots about eight inches across with medicine, and serve this to the men assembled in the square. He has already given instructions what order to observe and who are not to be served until the last because they have touched a dead body or for any other reason. The warm pasa is given first and then the cold miko hoyanídja. The miko and the other occupants of the central section of the Chiefs' bed are served first, then those at the south end right down to the Bird clan, then the henihálgi at the north end of the Chiefs' bed, then the tàstànàgis and ímalas in turn, i. e., those in the Warriors' bed from west to east, then those in the south bed from west to east, and finally those in the east bed from south to north. All those in the back seats come to the front unless some have to wait because they have dug a grave or something of the sort. The waiters drink last. Those who had eaten roasting ears of the same season already had to wait for their medicine until the others were through. Meanwhile a youth has been sent out after a pot of wormseed which is placed in front of the hilis-haya and as soon as the other medicines have been taken he blows into it. Each person then takes a little of it, chews some, and smears some on his body. They say this is 'to wash the head with.' Finally they go down to the creek headed by the miko and dive beneath the water four times. This ends the busk.

"In the morning while the above ceremony is taking place the boys are again summoned and sent for miko hoyanídja and the ten medicines used in the stomp dance. They take their busk medicine, which has been left for them on the bed of the henihálgi, when they come back. The stomp dance medicine is placed near the fire and taken there and they dance the stomp dance all that night until dawn.

"Next day the people lounge around, sleep, or play ball if they want to, but all come in that night for another jolly dance. On that morning thay have broken their fast. During this day a council is also held, and the miko sends word to the tástánágis that there will be a hunt next day, so all come up in the morning prepared for it. After the third drum beat all must be ready with their horses, and then they go out to some place where they think there will be good hunting. If they kill anything they leave it at the end of the Heníhas' bed; if they are unsuccessful, they say to the head tástánági 'We did not get anything,' and he reports to the miko.

"Next morning a piece of beef is brought; the hilis-haya blows upon and conjures this and puts it into the very center of the fire. Presumably this is to purify the people and insure them health, and also to feed the fire or some being in or through it. About noon the women dance in the same order as before, and this is also a day of feasting. The day after they fast all day, take their medicine as in the stomp dance, and dance all night. Before day the head tástánági addresses them telling them to behave well, that they have had a good time together and must not feel disturbed if their property has become injured during their absence. The miko then tells them to meet at such and such a time when the moon is at such and such a place, and they all go home.

"The above is an account of the later form of the busk at Tukabahchee, but in earlier days it was amplified in several particulars. The older form was identical with the above up to the appearance of the copper shields. From there it proceeds differently. The shields are carried out just at daylight by a squad of youths including one of the isti-átcagágis and one of the heníhas, or an even number of each—under the direction of the youths' captain. They proceed two at a time, those in advance each carrying a brass shield, and those behind each one of the pointed copper objects until there is a long procession. Proceeding to the creek before the fire is made they wash and scour them and carry them back. Then they hand them to the miko who lays them down in front of the hilis-haya. In addition to the regular pots of miko hoyanídja four others are conjured, after which the heníhas carry one to each bed and put it up in the center inside overhead. Then all are told to go and see about their horses, attend to other necessary duties, and come back again. A number of the isti-àtcagàgi remain, however. Meanwhile the boys have been sent out to get the àsi, which two men are appointed to parch. Then eight men come out and the miko has strings of beads put on the necks of four of them, who upon receiving these go back to their seats. A henīha gets the àsi and lays it down by the other medicines. The àsi looks like red haw. It is put into a pot and one of the boys appointed to do the parching stands on each side. Each holds a long paddle and stirs slowly. There is no water in the medicine until it is entirely parched, when water is poured into the pot to fill it up. It is then dipped up and strained back into the same pot through a basket strainer. All this is done with a regular rhythmic motion, and two men lying in the center of the east bed, an isti-àtcagàgi and a Panther, sing a slow, doleful song and shake their old gourds.

"It is now getting on toward noon. While the parching is proceeding the leader of the men who are going to carry the shields gets out near the medicine house and whoops twice. Then the eight men previously summoned, four of whom have probably returned their beads to the miko by this time, go out into the square and form two lines of four each extending from north to south on each side of the fire, facing the fire and with two leaders at the south end. The miko's henīha and another then go and fill their gourds or little pots with àsi which they then carry to the benches, and serve all those entitled to receive it, beginning with the miko and the other principal men. Each henīha crosses to the man immediately opposite to the one that his companion faces. The hilis-haya meanwhile is between the two lines near the fire. When the man who is served raises the pot to his lips the waiter shouts 'hwa-u-u-u' (the yahola cry), extending the sound as long as he can hold his breath, and when he is through the other takes a sip, spits it out, and hands the pot back to the waiter who then proceeds to the next man. After they have been round, what is left is taken to the hilis-haya. The hilis-haya and the old tàstànàgi (tcilaleiga?) have ladles with which they dip out the rest of the medicine until it is all gone, a fact which each announces. Then more àsi is parched and the man near the medicine house shouts two times more. This medicine is drunk like the first, and then the word is given to hurry, upon which the two men who have been singing and shaking their rattles run out toward the man in charge of the shields and the three pass around the tàdjo mound and back into the square on a 'dog-trot.' Then the miko takes the shields and plates and distributes them to the eight tàstànàgis who stand in line to receive them. The leader of the imała làbotcki orders them out, and each goes and gets a cane with a feather on the end of it. The two men who had lain in the northeast bed singing dance slowly out of the north entrance, round the tádjo mound and in again at the west entrance while the warriors and younger men dance round and round them faster all the way. They make this circuit four times, and the warriors and young men dance until the two old men have taken their seats. This dance is called the 'long dance' or the 'long whoop.' The feathers are fastened upon the canes used at this time by members of the Bird clan who have received orders that morning from the tálsá miko. The eagle feathers are placed near the kosi miko in the Beaver bed, and crane feathers at the end of the bed of the Bird clan. After that all retire until the evening.

"That evening the eight waiters start out at the northwest (or west) exit shouting 'yuayux,' the last man saying at intervals 'wátágu' (or natágu'?). They go all the way round on the outside until they come to the northeast bed and say 'I found nothing, I found nothing.' Then the isti-átcagági in that bed, who have set out a little gift of tobacco for them, shout 'hitci laiktci'' ('here is tobacco'). They repeat the same performance at each bed, and they make the circuit four times in all. They are called the 'tobacco beggars' and act as if they were spies or guards. Those fasting eat nothing and touch no women or anybody and the speaker gives the word to keep silence. That day is their 'sabbath.'

"Orders are issued that all the men return to the grounds before night, and there is a men's stomp dance that night to which no women are admitted. First they will perhaps dance 'the long dance,' with the feathers but without the shields. The shields lie on the bed of sand prepared for them all day until the morning of the day on which meat is put into the fire when they are returned to their usual place. During this time outsiders may look in from beyond the limits but none may come inside. Very early next morning a man is heard coming from the eastward whooping in the distance. By sunrise he gets behind the southwest bed and enters by the south entry. This is the itci yahola, who wears beads, leggings, a fancy hatchet, and four tufts of hair, like scalps, on 'the rim of a cap.' While he dances the tcukoleidji (women leaders) sing for him, beginning before he enters. These tcukoleidji used to sit in the Alligator bed at this time, but, the Alligator clan having died out, they were later in the Panthers' bed. While this man is dancing the warriors, assembled by command back of the Warriors' bed, divide into two parties, get out bows and arrows and pistols and act as if they are going to fight. Then the women and the two old men who sang when the ási was being parched move out to the tádjo mound, stopping a few minutes at the Alligator bed on the way, and singing all the time. The itci yahola dances around with his scalp headdress and tomahawk; he approaches in this way the north entrance where he is met by two other men, one of whom carries a gun. They and the two men on the tádjo mound sing responsively for a while. Meanwhile an image made of weeds has been placed half way between the tádjo and the north entrance, and when the singing is finished the man with the gun shoots at it and the one with the tomahawk runs up to it and pretends to scalp it. Upon this all the warriors (including the tcukoleidji) rush in together, first around the tádjo and then into the square, part dancing round in the usual manner and part in reverse, shooting off their guns and making a great noise. Then they all stampede down the hill to the creek and all are supposed to dive into the creek four times, though usually the women merely dash the water into their faces. This is the 'gun dance.' Then they (the tcukoleidji) will run back and catch some visitors and make them carry a log or something of the kind. There were eight or ten tcukoleidji, two being leaders. This ceremony is finished early in the day, and during the remainder of the day they lie about and rest. In the evening they have a little fun by dancing the dumpling dance, using the feathered sticks that were employed before, some having eagle feathers and some crane feathers.

"That same night orders are given to go hunting on the following morning. The men remain inside of the grounds every night; they may eat fresh sofki, fresh bread or honey or molasses, but no meat until the fourth morning. The morning after the gun dance they go hunting and the morning after that the meat is put into the fire as already related. This finishes the conjuring of the fire. Then the wormseed is used, they bathe in the creek, and 'the busk is destroyed.'

"The women dance that night and then they dance the 'old dance,' after which the men attend to their horses, and do any other necessary work. Next day they fast all day and have a stomp dance at night, and the morning following the miko makes them an address, tells them to be good, etc., and says 'When the moon is so and so you will hear from me.' Then they eat breakfast and go home.

"If any of the warriors does not come to the busk they afterwards send to exact a fine from him, or, if he is within reach, the first day they go out hunting they go and see what they can get from him. If a man stayed away from the busk persistently his seat might be declared vacant and a young man selected to fill it. This regulation applied to the other Creek towns as well. In later times whiskey was not allowed on the grounds and if any one brought it he was subject to a severe fine.

"Anciently two orderlies were sent around among the camps to see whether any of the young men who should be fasting had broken the bounds and gone off into the woods to sleep or to have intercourse with women." According to my informant such offenders were almost always found out.

Some say that anciently the Tukabahchee had to busk before all other Creek towns. As we have seen, Atasi, Liwahali, and Laplako used to go to Tukabahchee in later times to get their medicine; the Kealedji only sent for fire and returned the next morning while the rest remained and finished the busk with the Tukabahchee. It is said that Alabama and Hilibi were formerly attached in the same manner but became separated in course of time. In the same way Coweta and Eufaula are said to have busked together at one time.[51] Any stranger who once took medicine at Tukabahchee had to take it there for four successive years before he could take it anywhere else. These statements were made by a very old Indian, but for the most part they represent not an ancient condition but a later readjustment, after some of these towns had begun to fall off in numbers.

Earlier descriptions of the Tukabahchee busk, mostly confirmatory of the above though showing certain variations, are given by Stiggins and Hitchcock, the latter apparently mainly on the authority of James Islands. Stiggins says:

"I have made frequent mention of their celebration of the anniversary of the New Corn Crop, called by them *Booske tah*, as much as to say 'sacred purifying,' which is the only thing wherein I ever saw them act as though they paid adoration to the all supreme. They seem even when they are preparing to go to the festival to solemnize their minds and actions as a devout person would enter a church to worship, and it is evident that originally it must have had great weight even in their political movements, for it will, after its celebration, stop the proceedings against any offender where life and death is not concerned, and stealing is not exempted. All other misdemeanors pass into oblivion, and a new score is begun for the ensuing festival. The Cowassawdays hold one festival more than the rest of the nation as they annually celebrate the coming of the new crop of beans with the same ceremonies as they do the festival of corn.[52] I have made a small digression from the point in [detailing] the order of their festival. I shall proceed to it in as accurate a manner as I can by saying that when the head men of a town see that the town or public corn is full in the ear and fit for use they set a day and inform the town people when the sacred festival is to commence.

"Before the day arrives they nominate some of their *emathlahs*, which word means 'gone at his bidding,' to boil their physic that they drink and bathe in in order to purify themselves, and of their most respectable chiefs they nominate three to officiate in the duties of

---

[51] Yet, according to another informant, the Eufaula formerly got their fire from Kealedji.
[52] Could this be the same as that held to "sanctify the mulberries?" (See p. 550.)

the time as sacred priests or doctors. They then send some of the *emathlahs,* to gather a bush that acts as a quick and powerful emetic; they call it *micco ho yan ejah.* It is a 'kings cathartic.' They break enough to last the festival out. The bush is very much like the low myrtle bush in appearance but bears no berries. When the appointed festival day arrives all the town people put out their fires and repair to the town house or square when they commence the sacred festival. They have particular songs and dances for it; they dance during the festival at intervals. Their singers are generally some men of eminence invited from some other town as proficient singers, and they take it as a mark of distinction to receive an invitation for that purpose. After all have congregated they select men to boil physic, and those nominated to officiate as sacred men make a fire out of the public way so that they may not be polluted by the touch of an unpurified person during their strict penance, as they account their person sacred during their sacred and purified office. They proceed to boil their *a wo teach caw* [sawàtcka] which is an emetic. After it is thoroughly boiled the three men selected for the sacred office take it after it is put into large cooling pans of clay manufactory, and prepare it for drinking and bathing. Each man takes a pan and sets it before him and commences the process of cooling, having his head covered over and the joint of a cane in his hand. During the time they each sing a song of requests and thanks in a low under voice to the giver or taker of breath called *saw ga emisse.* In every interval the singer sticks his cane joint into the pan of *awa teach caw* and blows the virtue of said song of requests into the pan of physic in a most solemn manner, so that therewith it might operate in good to them that drink thereof. It is a quick and rapid emetic and drank for that purpose by all the men, and nearly all the women wash their children with it; the Creek Indians have no variation in their annual celebration of the new crop of corn, having particular songs and dances for the festive purpose. The commemoration in every town holds two days in the minor village towns, not including the first day. The Tuckabahchee town being the metropolis of the nation has a variety of show in their solemn feast; they continue it for six days. It is attended always by a large congregation who resort there to see and be seen.

" During their six days of *Boos ke tah* neither those set apart for doctoring or physic making, nor such as are appointed to show the strict rule or penance necessary on the occasion, make use of anything to eat or drink but the consecrated emetic of which they take profusely every day of the festival. They neither speak to nor touch a woman during said time as such a procedure would inevitably ruin their thanksgiving song, and instead of a blessing involve destruction, not only to the offender but to the community at large; nor will they shake hands with nor touch an unpurified friend during the time of their officiating. The whole festival is conducted with a grave, superstitious solemnity to the last day. On the last day they take out and exhibit the afore-mentioned six brass or breast plates. They are carried around by three men, one in each hand, in that day's dance. With much superstitious awe said plates are kept under the care of two men always, and after their exhibition in the dances they are laid in the depository, which is under the seats that uphold the mats that the kings sit on, in their part of the council square. It is said that three of said brass plates have hieroglyphic signs on them, whilst others say that they could trace Hebrew characters in a circle in the central part of the three oval ones. As they are scoured and burnished every year before they are exhibited no doubt the characters are nearly defaced. Their traditional account of how they came by them is that they were thrown or handed down by the *Giver or Taker of Breath,* viz. *Saw ga Emisse,* with an assurance to them that so long as they used them undefiled in their festivals no people could divest them of their festival ceremonies or country. On the same day they exhibit their manner of attack in warfare; several effigies are brought and placed about in the square to be attacked in a hostile manner by men appointed for the purpose, who, to show their skill in coming on their enemy by stealth, come on the effigies with all imaginable caution as though unperceived by them as an enemy. When they get near the square they all at once raise the war scream and charge on them, shoot, tomahawk, and scalp them, and though pursued by others they make their escape as they would in actual attack. As many have passed their time fasting it is necessary to eat of the new corn, and as all things in their political life have a new beginning, it is necessary to have new fire with which to cook their corn and other eatables, so that morning four men are appointed to the duty. Each takes a block with a small incision in it and a round stick and apply it in the indenture of the block and roll it to and fro in the palms of their hands until it takes fire by the friction. There is great expression of joy when the new fire is made; every family in the town and even adjacent townspeople take the new fire home to use in cooking during that year.

"In the course of the festival and usually at night in intervals for rest the young men are divested of their given name that they had from infancy and invested with what is called a war name by which they are known for the rest of their lives. It is done thus. Previous to the ceremony of naming the name that he is thereafter to assume is intimated to the young man by one of the kings or warriors, for either can give names. When the time arrives for the ceremony one of the kings or warriors rises from his seat and calls the name in a shrill, long tone of voice. At the call the young man rises, picks up the war club or mallet called by them *attussa* and goes forth to him, when he informs the new man that he is now named as other men and he now can assume the manners and customs of other men. He then puts a feather on his head and when that is done the newly dubbed man raises his war club above his head, starts a long whoop, and runs round in a circle to the place from which he started and when he stops he cries 'youh youh.' From that time on he is a man with a name. After the *Boos ke tah* it is known that all light offenses are past into oblivion." [53]

Hitchcock's account runs thus:

"At the season of green corn, usually in July, the chiefs of the town meet and have a talk with their people about the Green Corn Dance. At this meeting they give orders to make the pots and other utensils needed, except those which are sacred. Some of the sacred utensils have been handed down [from] time immemorial. They meet again in seven days, again four days afterwards, and then again in two days. At these several meetings they give orders for preparations, appoint persons to procure wood, others to procure cane, etc., etc. At the fourth meeting they give out the 'broken days' for the Busk, seven from the day they give notice, or six not counting the day when the notice is given.

"All persons on the fifth night are ordered to encamp in the vicinity of the Square. On the sixth day all the women, dressed in full costume loaded with ornaments, dance for about three hours in the middle of the day. There are men appointed to watch them and if anyone leaves the dance without a good excuse, as sickness or other sufficient cause, she is deprived of her ornaments which are confiscated and she does not return. A certain number of women are appointed to conduct the dance and these are not allowed to eat until after the dance is over and they have bathed in the branch or creek. Before the dance these conductors are covered with what is called medicine, some sacred preparation, and this must be washed off before they can eat. The night of the day on which the women dance the men and women dance together. This is a friendly, familiar dance without particular preparation or ceremony. The day following, that is the sixth day [but the first of the regular ceremonial days], is a sacred day and the men fast all day, and during the day they take a medicine prepared from an herb that operates like a powerful emetic. On this day, the sixth, the sacred fire is made in a small house in a corner of the Square. The twelve persons appointed for this purpose remain all of the preceding night in the square and at early dawn[54] they commence a frictional process, rub-

[53] Stiggins, Ms.
[54] Elsewhere he says "at the crowing of the cock in the morning."

bing a piece of cane in decayed wood with great velocity until the wood ignites. Sometimes it requires many hours for this.[55] The persons appointed for the purpose then prepare, over the fire, the medicine (emetic) with which the men cleanse themselves. During the day only those who take this medicine and those having duties there by appointment are allowed to enter the square.

"On the same day (the sixth) the sacred plates and other holy utensils are taken by persons appointed for the purpose from the places where they have been preserved, unseen by human eyes, for a twelve month, they thoroughly scour and clean them, and about one o'clock they are brought into the square. These utensils are regarded as presents from the Great Spirit. They are brought into the square with great state and ceremony. The persons bearing them are preceded by two men provided with cocoanut shells which they rattle continually, the men singing all the time, and they are followed by others with long reeds from the ends of which white feathers stream in the wind. The whole procession dances into the square and around it four times and then passes outside and dances around another spot four times. Then they again enter the square repeating the dance in and out four times. After this the sacred pieces are delivered over to the King (Micco) and after fasting all day and all night and dancing all night [on the second day of the ceremony], they dance the War Dance. For this dance there are two men selected called the head warriors. These two come into the square just before day unclothed except for a piece of stroud, but they are painted and covered with ornaments and carry a pouch for their pipe and tobacco. There are a number of women selected to assist the men in singing the war song for the two men to dance after around the square, or the ring in the center of the square. During the dancing two separate parties are selected and dressed like the two warriors except that they have shot pouches and rifles, and effigies are prepared and set up outside of the square to represent enemies surmounted with scalps, generally representing one woman and two men. The warriors approach in the Indian mode of advancing to battle by stealthily crawling behind such objects as make the best screens. (During all this time the two warriors are dancing inside of the square.)

"There are spies out who discover the approach of the two parties about to surround the effigies, and they go to the corner of the square and give notice to the two warriors that their friends in two parties are about to surround their enemies, the effigies. As soon as this is done a man rushes out beating a drum, and at the tap of the drum the head warriors come out of the square, each with an aid, and all four take up a position resting upon one knee, the chiefs with the

---

[55] Elsewhere he says "all the morning and until afternoon."

tomahawks and their aids with rifles presented towards the effigies.
While in that position they sing a very solemn war song which is
answered in a chorus by their friends, the two parties of warriors.
During the singing, the women, who were appointed to sing in the
square, pass to a heap of earth previously thrown up for the purpose
and are joined by their female friends for the purpose of welcoming
their husbands and brothers returned from war. As soon as the
women are assembled the head warriors give orders to advance.
They take the lead themselves and scalp the effigies, and the two
parties meet over the effigies as soon as they are scalped and fire their
rifles at will accompanied with an uproar of whooping and yelling.
They then pass around the hill where the women are and while the
women sing and the men dance, whoop and yell, loading and firing
their rifles. After dancing around their women for some time the
men enter, firing the guns and rejoicing and dance around the
square four times. They then terminate the ceremony for that day,
those who have been dancing going to the branch and bathing.
After this they return to the square and break their fast by eating
green corn without limit with every other kind of vegetable—pump-
kins, water melons, etc—but no meat nor salt. This occurs about
8 or 9 o'clock in the morning and the remaining portion of the day
is devoted to rest as also the night following, except that some may
choose to dance for amusement.

"It is a rule that if, before the Green Corn Dance, any person
has eaten green corn or even the food cooked at the fire where corn
has been roasted or otherwise prepared for food he is not allowed to
participate in the dance or Busk. All who participate in the ceremony are required to clear away the fire and ashes from their domestic
hearths and rekindle it with fire which has been made at the square.
All who participate in the Busk and take the medicine are obliged
for four days to sleep at the square every night and are not allowed
to be with their wives. On the third day of the Busk the men
dance with the plates and then go out with their rifles to kill deer,
returning early in the afternoon (about 2 o'clock) with meat. They
eat no meat this day, however, but satiate their appetite with sofkee,
etc. The night is passed in dancing and sleeping according to their
pleasure, the women not being present. On the fourth day the meat
is prepared with salt and eaten for breakfast. After breakfast the
women dance in the square, the men merely looking on. Until this
day those who have eaten salt are not allowed to touch the ones
engaged in the ceremony, who do not, until the fourth day, touch
salt themselves. Toward the close of the day the men and women
dance what is called the bison dance. The men wear only the
stroud except that they add bushes and other means of assimilating
their appearance to that of animals. They bend half forward and

while dancing imitate the bellowing of bison. The women have terrapin shells loaded with peas and fastened to strips of leather in rows of three or four tied below their knees. The night of the fourth day the men and women dance together and then disperse to their homes except certain persons appointed for the purpose who remain at the square and sleep there three or four nights. After dancing around the plates on the third day, they deposit the latter in their appointed place of safety where they remain carefully protected until required the next year.

"During the ceremony . . . the young men frequently engage in a ball play or other amusement and . . . everything wears the appearance of rejoicing and gladness, and thanksgiving for the blessings of a plentiful promise of the productions of the earth." [56]

To these may be added an account of a visit to the Tukabahchee busk of July, 1917, by Mr. G. W. Grayson, late chief of the Creek Nation, found among his papers and copied by the writer with the kind permission of Mr. Grayson's family. Unfortunately, one page of the manuscript is missing. I have found it necessary to make a few changes in the wording for the sake of smoothness. The most important contribution contained in this narrative is the insight it gives into the customs observed in receiving a guest from a friendly town. A stray note informs us, on the authority of one of the oldest men in Tukabahchee, that the Power Above who had instituted the ceremony said, "You shall not call my name openly in the congregation; if you do, it will not be well with you."

"[I] arrived at Tuckabatchee Busk ground on July 27, 1917, while the women, twenty-six in number, were dancing. Most of them were apparently of middle age and probably mothers of families. They appeared to be very respectable women and were adorned with long wide ribbons of silk flowing gorgeously from their heads, very much like the women whom we saw some five years ago in the dances of this kind as then conducted by the Okfuskeys near the present town of Eufaula.

"After the women had executed several rounds, they were required to surrender their vttussa vhake ['like war-clubs,' little wooden sticks carved in a manner supposed to resemble the forms of the ancient war-clubs], when the men engaged in the Old dance (punka vcale) mixed up with the women in their ribbons and finery. One round of this was danced and that ended the exercises. At night the people danced until about 10 o'clock and recessed until the morrow.

(Here a page is missing.)

". . . Since last night the buskers have been fasting and must continue it all this day [July 28], and tonight and until tomorrow morning when they will be permitted to partake of food. It is with

---

[56] Hitchcock, Ms. notes.

regret that they admit that the correct practices of the Busk as they obtained in the olden days are not now correctly known to any of the members. This fact became painfully evident some years ago when the old men counseled together over the subject and decided that they would hereafter confine the exercises of the Busk to what is known as the 'Boy's Fast' (Chebunuckochee im Pusketa), since no member appears able to instruct in or conduct correctly the proper exercises for the adults, while there were many who could conduct the Boy's Fast correctly. So all that we can now see of the Busk is what is known as the Boy's Fast.

"The copper or brass plates are so sacred, and their exposure and handling by incompetent hands so liable to be attended by dire consequences, that we cannot get a view of them. It appears that the town has no medicine men who are sufficiently educated in the mysteries to uncover and handle them. The tradition respecting these plates is that when the Town becomes unable to handle them properly, they are to be surrendered to the Shawnees, and the old man Sardy says they may come now and demand them any year.

"Late this evening I was informed that since the Cowetas, of which I am a member, have ever been the 'big friend' of the Tuckabatchees, and I, a Coweta, though unknown to the majority of the Buskers, had paid them a visit the town owed me a formal reception in keeping with the ancient custom of the respective towns which they desired should be tendered me in accordance with that custom. It transpired, however, that no one save the old gentleman Conchart Emarthla, by whom I had been entertained all day at his camp, knew anything of the ancient customs to be observed at such receptions, and he was lying prone on his back in his camp and in misery from muscular rheumatism. He was solicited by several different messengers from the town chief, sent at several separate times, to go to the dance circle and conduct the reception ceremony, which, despite his ailment, and in deference to me, he was willing to do provided he could be conveyed from his camp to the dance circle. After a number of consultations on the subject, during which the people were busily engaged in the common stomp dance in the square near by, it was decided that the old gentleman should be conveyed in his daughter's $1,600 automobile, standing a few steps from his camp. I accompanied him in the automobile, which his son drove for us, and on the way to the square he instructed me to remain in the auto while he went to confer with the authorities on the subject, after which a messenger would soon be sent to conduct me in as was customary on such occasions. I was to follow him and, when near the seats, say in a voice clearly audible to the assembly, 'I have arrived.'

"Accordingly, on our arrival at the square the old gentleman went in and after some little delay delivered a characteristic, old-

fashioned speech treating in part of the ancient friendship subsist-
ing between the Tuckabatchees and Cowetas. He told the audience
that one of the Cowetas had arrived and that he should be received
with all those formalities 'that it was the custom of our forefathers to
observe on such occasions in times past.' The old gentleman, in
short, delivered a splendid address in the ancient manner, the kind
that was once so common with public speakers among the Creeks.
After this address, I was conducted into the circle by a special messenger. When I came before the men, who were disposed on seats
made of logs, I exclaimed as I had been previously instructed, 'I
have arrived.' The old man then instructed the audience as to the
order of the hand shaking that was now to be performed. After the
hand-shaking I exchanged small bits of 'Star' tobacco—a brand
of the manufactured weed much in vogue at this time with chewers
of tobacco—with each of the audience, and when we finished the
proceeding the pockets of my coat were well loaded with these bits
of tobacco. When we were through with this performance, the old
gentleman at whose side I sat called up Arbeca Micco, a son of Geo.
Long deceased, and, informing him that I was of his own, the Tiger,
clan, directed him to conduct me to a seat among the members of
his clan where I could be with the other Tigers. This he did and I
sat conversing with the Tigers, while the dance was going on, for
about an hour, when I retired to my pallet in a tent assigned to me
by John Harjo at his camp. The dance was continued until daylight
Sunday morning.

"Sunday, July 29th, 1917.—I arose quite early this morning and
after breakfast went out to the dance circle where a few men were
lying about on the ground and on the old wooden log seats asleep
and a few others were sitting in small groups conversing lazily, though
much fatigued by the exercises of the all night dance. The only
sight that I got was a better view of the United States flag, which
floated from a staff near the town chief's seat. This flag the Indians
call in their language A-book-he Tca-te ["red flag"]. I also saw
the old pine box, about 30 inches square I should judge, sitting on
the log seats provided for the chiefs' shed, in which I was informed
were inclosed the Brass or Copper plates of which we have so often
heard."

If two families lived a long way from their own busk grounds but
near each other's, they sometimes swapped duties, each going to the
nearer ground. Such swapping usually took place only between
towns in the same fire clan but Cook has known of such an exchange between Tulsa and Tukabahchee Indians. If a man had
married outside his town, he was obliged to attend the busk in his
wife's town as well as the one in his own, but he could not dance at
the former. If he stayed away from the busk of his wife's people, he

would be fined a sum amounting, in later times, to something like
$10, and if he refused to pay his horse would be carried off.

The Tukabahchee busk proper lasted theoretically eight days, two
more than the number given by Stiggins, and this number may be
made out if we include the day of assembly and preparation
and the day when the people separated to go home. Anciently
the busks of Coweta, Kasihta, Kealedji, and perhaps some of
the other larger towns were of eight days also, but those of
the smaller towns were of four days' duration only, and this difference existed as far back as the time of Hawkins, at the end of the
eighteenth century.[57] It is plain from the description of the Tukabahchee busk that it really consisted of a repetition of the same
thing twice. First there is a day for arranging the preliminaries,
placing visitors, etc., next a day of feasting, then a day of fasting,
then a day of relaxation. Then comes a day of hunting correspond-
ing to the day of preparation, a second day of feasting, a second day
of fasting, and finally a day when they dispersed. The same idea of
repetition by fours, or of the division of the long busk into two
periods of four days each, is in evidence in the other accounts which
we have of the long form, but the various elements are not always
reckoned in the same manner nor do they occur in the same invariable
sequence. The earliest account of a Creek eight-day busk which
attempts to present the happenings day by day is that of Hawkins,
which has been frequently quoted. As it is important to compare
this with the accounts already given it is subjoined.

"*First Day.*—In the morning, the warriors clean the yard of the
square, and sprinkle white sand, when the a-cee (decoction of the
cassine yupon) is made. The fire-maker makes the fire as early in
the morning as he can, by friction. The warriors cut and bring into
the square, four logs, as long each as a man can cover by extending
his two arms; these are placed in the centre of the square, end to end,
forming a cross, the outer ends pointed to the cardinal points; in
the centre of the cross, the new fire is made. During the first four
days, they burn out these four logs.

"The pin-e-bun-gau, (turkey dance,) is danced by the women of
the turkey tribe; and while they are dancing the possau is brewed.
This is a powerful emetic. The possau is drank from twelve o'clock
to the middle of the afternoon. After this, the Toc-co-yule-gau
[tokyûlga] (tadpole,) is danced by four men and four women. (In
the evening, the men dance E-ne-hou-bun-gau [heníha obánga], the
dance of the people second in command.) This they dance till
daylight.

[57] That the eight-day busk was anciently more general is indicated, however, by Eakins's statement
that it "formerly embraced a period of eight days, but now a period of four days." (Schoolcraft, Ind.
Tribes, vol. I, p. 272.)

"*Second Day.*—This day, about ten o'clock, the women dance Its-ho-bun-dau [Itcha obánga] (gun-dance).[58] After twelve, the men go to the new fire, take some of the ashes, rub them on the chin, neck and belly, and jump head foremost into the river, and they return into the square. The women having prepared the new corn for the feast, the men take some of it and rub it between their hands, then on their faces and breasts, and then they feast.

"*Third Day.*—The men sit in the square.

"*Fourth Day.*—The women go early in the morning and get the new fire, clean out their hearths, sprinkle them with sand, and make their fires. The men finish burning out the first four logs, and they take ashes, rub them on their chin, neck and belly, and they go into the water. This day they eat salt, and they dance Obengauchapco [Obánga tcápko] (the long dance).

"*Fifth Day.*—They get four new logs, and place them as on the first day, and they drink a-cee, a strong decoction of the cassine yupon.

"*Sixth Day.*—They remain in the square.

"*Seventh Day.*—Is spent in like manner as the sixth.

"*Eighth Day.*—They get two large pots, and their physic plants, 1st. Mic-co-ho-yon-e-juh [miko hoyanídja]. 2. Toloh. 3. A-che-nau [atcīna]. 4. Cup-pau-pos-cau [kápapaska]. 5. Chu-lis-sau, the roots. 6. Tuck-thlau-lus-te [tokła lasti]. 7. Tote-cul-hil-lis-se-wau [totka hiliswa]. 8. Chofeinsuck-cau-fuck-au [tcufi insákofáká].[59] 9. Cho-fe-mus-see. 10. Hil-lis-hut-ke [hilis hátki]. 11. To-te cuh chooc-his-see. 12. Welau-nuh [wīláná]. 13. Oak-chon-utch-co [ok-tcanitcka]. 14. Co-hal-le-wau-gee [koha liwagi, young soft cane]. These are all put into the pots and beat up with water. The chemists (E-lic-chul-gee [Aliktcálgi], called by the traders physic makers,) they blow in it through a small reed, and then it is drank by the men, and rubbed over their joints till the afternoon.

"They collect old corn cobs and pine burs, put them into a pot, and burn them to ashes. Four virgins who have never had their menses, bring ashes from their houses, put them in the pot and stir all together. The men take white clay and mix it with water in two pans. One pan of the clay and one of the ashes, are carried to the cabin of the Mic-co, and the other two to that of the warriors. They then rub themselves with the clay and ashes. Two men appointed to that office, bring some flowers of tobacco of a small kind, (Itch-au-chu-le-puc-pug-gee [Hitci atculi pákpági] or, as the name imports, the old man's tobacco, which was prepared on the first day, and put in a pan on the cabin of the Mic-co, and they give a little of it to every one present.

---

[58] Hawkins has made an error here on account of the close resemblance of two words. Gun is i'tca, but this is itcha' and the dance is usually called a "women's dance."

[59] This is called "buck bush" in English. The Creek word means "rabbit's carrying-basket string."

"The Micco and counsellors then go four times round the fire, and every time they face the east, they throw some of the flowers into the fire. They then go and stand to the west. The warriors then repeat the same ceremony.

"A cane is stuck up at the cabin of the Mic-co with two white feathers in the end of it. One of the Fish tribe, (Thlot-lo-ul-gee [Lȧlogȧlgi],) takes it just as the sun goes down, and goes off toward the river, all following him. When he gets half way to the river, he gives the death whoop; this whoop he repeats four times, between the square and the water's edge. Here they all place themselves as thick as they can stand, near the edge of the water. He sticks up the cane at the water's edge, and they all put a grain of the old man's tobacco on their heads, and in each ear. Then, at a signal given, four different times, they throw some into the river, and every man at a like signal plunges into the river, and picks up four stones from the bottom. With these they cross themselves on their breats four times, each time throwing a stone into the river, and giving the death whoop; they then wash themselves, take up the cane and feathers, return and stick it up in the square, and visit through the town. At night they dance O-bun-gau Haujo [Obȧngȧ hadjo], (mad dance,) and this finishes the ceremony." [60]

It is to be noticed that four logs are burned up on the first four days, at the end of which time the men rub ashes upon their bodies and go into the water to bathe, and that in the second period of four days the same thing is repeated except that clay is added to the ashes. The division into two periods is further accentuated by the use of pasa on the first day of the first period and the use of the miko hoyanȋdja and the other medicines, the adilō'ga, on the last day of the last period. It is also to be observed that ȧsi was drunk early on the first and fifth days. This separate use of the two medicines is of course a considerable variation from the later usage, and there are in fact many differences. Among these it may be noted that the yard was cleaned on the first day of the busk and not at some previous time as is now customary. Next that the new fire was made on the very first day instead of the fasting day, but the women did not clean out their hearths and relight them until the fourth day, whereas they do it now —or did some years back—immediately after the kindling. Since the Turkey women danced the turkey dance on the morning of the first day, just before the pasa was drunk, and women participated in the tadpole dance right afterward, it would appear that the square was not shut off when this medicine was taken or if it was it was only for a few hours, "from twelve o'clock to the middle of the afternoon." It is to be noted that the men rubbed themselves with ashes and jumped into the river on the second day as well as the fourth and

[60] Ga. Hist. Soc. Colls., vol. III, pp. 75-78.

eighth. This would suggest three periods of fasting instead of two, but Hawkins unfortunately does not tell us just when the men fasted and when they were shut up within the bounds of the square. On the third, sixth, and seventh days we are told that the men sat in the square but we do not know whether they were fasting or lounging. At least they appear not to have been taking the medicine at that time. The conjuration with native tobacco was probably, as we know it to have been in later times, to keep away ghosts. I do not know what the ceremonial with the river pebbles may have signified. It will be noticed that this ceremony closed as usual with the mad or drunken dance.

Hodgson gives a short reference to a busk, probably the Kasihta busk, on the authority of a white trader who had been in the Creek Nation 15 years.

"Before the corn turns yellow, the inhabitants of each town or district assemble; and a certain number enter the streets of what is more properly called the town, with the war-whoop and savage yells, firing their arrows in the air, and going several times around the pole. They then take emetics, and fast two days; dancing round the pole a great part of the night. All the fires in the township are then extinguished, and the hearths cleared, and new fires kindled by rubbing two sticks. After this, they parch some of the new corn, and, feasting a little, disperse to their several homes. Many of the old Chiefs are of opinion, that their ancestors intended this ceremony as a thank-offering to the Supreme Being, for the fruits of the earth, and for success in hunting or in war."[61]

If Bartram's short account, which probably applies to the Atasi busk, is to be relied upon there were considerable differences between the busks of even the Upper Creek towns in his time. He says that they fasted and took medicine for three days, and on the fourth day lighted the new fire, prepared new corn and fruits, and had a feast followed by an all night dance. "This," he says, "continues three days, and the four following days they receive visits, and rejoice with their friends from neighboring towns, who have purified and prepared themselves." [62] If we reckon in all of the days given here this busk would extend to from 10 to 12 days, but the account of it is too fragmentary to be trusted very far. From an earlier statement of Bartram's it would seem that this town made an unusually clean sweep of its worn-out property before the ceremony. He says that "having previously provided themselves with new cloaths, new pots, pans, and other household utensils and furniture, they collect all their worn out clothes and other despicable things, sweep and cleanse their houses, squares, and the whole town, of their filth, which with all the remaining grain and other old pro-

---

visions, they cast together into one common heap, and consume it with fire."[63]

Milfort, however, says much the same, speaking perhaps particularly of Otciapofa. "Each year, in the month of August, they assemble by settlements (par habitation) to celebrate the harvest festival; then they renew all that they have used during the year which has just expired; the women break and shatter all their household utensils, and renew them."[64]

The four-day ceremony as recorded and observed by myself is very like the Tukabahchee ceremony cut in half, minus, of course, the shield ceremonial and in general stripped of much of the complication of the latter. The Eufaula ceremony always came in July and within recent years, instead of being determined by the moon, it has been fixed definitely on the 15th of July. The 13th is the day of assembly, the 14th the feast day, and the 16th the day when all separate. Thus the four are made out. I have seen part of this busk myself, but the following account from Jackson Lewis is reproduced by preference, since it gives the less corrupted ceremonial of an earlier period.

The first day of the ceremonial is, as we know, the day for assembling. "On the second day the women begin dancing about 4 p. m. They get through before dark and at dark the men and women dance together around the fire for from one to three hours. Then the men are informed by the chiefs that they must prepare to take the medicine on the morrow. The woman's dance is conducted always by the Hathagas (owners of the white); no other clans can have anything to do with it. While the women dance the chiefs send out men to cut four sticks of wood three or four feet long, which are brought in and prepared. Next morning all of the ashes of the previous fires are raked away and in the place which they occupied a quantity of new earth is deposited brought in from outside of the grounds. On this the fire-maker kindles a new fire made of four sticks of wood pointing to the four cardinal points. One person is detailed for the sole purpose of watching and keeping up the fire during the day on which the medicine is being taken. After the sun is fairly well up two persons are sent to dig up medicine roots and macerate them ready for treatment by the doctor. As the drinkers of the medicine exhaust the supply these two men bring up water to replace it. One of these belongs to the same clan as the town chief and outranks the other who is from the henihálgi, and is called his heniha.

"Any person can be detailed by the chiefs as replenisher of the fire. The maker of the fire, who is usually an old man well initiated into

[63] Bartram, Travels, p. 507.   [64] Milfort, Mém., p. 216.

the mysteries, puts the final medicine into the compound, sings a song over it, and blows into it through a cane. After this he sits still for a while thinking of what he is going to say and probably repeating a formula to himself. Then he again blows and again sits quiet, repeating this for some time, and finally he tells the people that it is ready for them. This medicine consists of mìko hoyanīdja, with which they combine wormseed. The ási or cassine is not now used. When all is ready the chiefs are informed of it and they first of all come up and take large potations. All those of the north bed partake first, facing the east as they drink; afterward the henihálgi, then the tástánágàlgi, and finally all others. A portion of the medicine is carried over to a place between the north and east beds and placed there for the women and children. As it is to ward off disease and misfortune they wet their faces and hands in it and wet the faces and hands of their children. The medicine is taken in this way four times during the day. No particular number of pots is prescribed. Formerly they were pots made of earthenware, but now barrels have taken their place. They are always so placed that the sun cannot shine on the liquid inside. It is usually drunk in large quantities and then vomited forth, but some who do not wish to vomit it out take small quantities of liquid and wash their faces and wêt their hands in it. About the third time the medicine has been taken the hathagàlgi gather a number of slender canes (here slender switches from the bottoms are used, 8 or 9 feet long). They kill a little white heron (fus hátki)—if they can kill a white crane it is better still—take the white feathers from it and tie them on the ends of the canes. The hathagàlgi do this and they also detail two persons to superintend the dance and see that it is properly conducted. The functions of these two men are indicated by canes three or four feet long with feathers tied to one end. The long switches are then distributed to all of the men who have been taking medicine. Bearing them they then engage in the dance known as tcitahaia, after which they take the medicine for the fourth time and then repair to the nearest water-hole to bathe. During all this time the grounds are marked off and made prohibited ground, and anyone not taking medicine may not go beyond the line marked off around it. The people taking medicine dare not come in contact with anyone who is not taking it. When these people have bathed and gotten back these prohibitions are removed. During the taking of the medicine the chief's interpreter speaks for him and lectures the people, the chief telling him what to say. This speaker is generally taken from the Potato clan. In his speech the chief counsels the people, especially the women, not to speak evilly of each other, to dwell in fellowship with all, and he counsels hospitality to all who have come to the busk. Many similar talks through the same interpreter are made during the busk. This lecturing is of very ancient origin. On the night of the 15th all of the people—men, women, and children—engage in "the all-night dance." This concludes the busk for the year.

"Long intervals elapse between the first and second and second and third drinkings which the chiefs make use of to select young men to receive new names. A person is selected by the chiefs to inform the youths, and he goes to each of them letting him know what is planned. At Eufaula the men are usually named in pairs, and one of the two must be a person who has already been named at some previous time. One person, or more than two, may, however, be named. After the youths have been informed the chief usually employs his interpreter to call these young men up, and he calls out the new name the youth is to bear twice in a long drawn out voice as if the youth were far away. The youth does not come until the second call. When he comes up they give him a bit of tobacco, but in very ancient times they presented him with a small piece of a scalp taken from the enemy. It is handed to him by the chief's interpreter, and, having received it, the youth waves it over the head of the chief, toward the roof of his cabin and says 'Yu yu' upon which all in the cabin reply 'Madō', thank you. Then he goes back to his seat."

If a man ate roasting ears before the busk no one would touch him or have anything to do with him. Such a person was given medicine last. At Hilibi if a person died during the busk they would fast, drink medicine, and dance all night and by the next noon take dinner as usual. They would do likewise if a man had gotten drunk. There is an indisposition to talk about sacred things, especially matters connected with the busk, unless one is fasting. One informant said "I can tell a little round the outside but not all for I have had my meals."

Swan gives the following account of a four-day busk on the authority of Alexander McGillivray, and it must therefore have been the ancient observance at Otciapofa:

"When corn is ripe, and the cassina or new black-drink has come to perfection, the busking begins on the morning of a day appointed by the priest, or fire-maker (as he is styled) of the town, and is celebrated for four days successively.

"On the morning of the first day, the priest, dressed in white leather moccasins and stockings, with a white dressed deerskin over his shoulders, repairs at break of day, unattended, to the square. His first business is to create the new fire, which he accomplishes with much labor by the friction of two dry sticks. After the fire is produced, four young men enter at the openings of the four corners of the square, each having a stick of wood for the new fire; they approach the new fire with much reverence, and place the ends of the wood they carry, in a very formal manner, to it.[64a] After the fire

---

[64a] Cf. pp. 561–562, 589.

is sufficiently kindled, four other young men come forward in the
same manner, each having a fair ear of new corn, which the priest
takes from them, and places with great solemnity in the fire, where
it is consumed.   Four young warriors then enter the square in the
manner before mentioned, each having some of the new cassina.   A
small part of it is given to the new fire by the priest, and the remainder is immediately parched and cooked for use.   During these
formalities, the priest is continually muttering some mysterious
jargon which nobody understands, nor is it proper for any inquiries
to be made on the subject; the people in general believe that he is
then communicating with the *great master of breath*.

"At this time, the warriors and others being assembled, they proceed to drink black-drink in their usual manner.   Some of the new
fire is next carried and left on the outside of the square, for public
use; and the women allowed to come and take it to their several
houses, which have the day before been cleaned, and decorated with
green boughs, for its reception; all the old fire in the town having
been previously extinguished, and the ashes swept clean away, to
make room for the new.   During this day, the women are suffered to
dance with the children on the outside of the square, but by no
means suffered to come into it.   The men keep entirely by themselves, and sleep in the square.

"The second day is devoted by the men to taking their war-
physic.   It is a strong decoction of the button snake-root, or sen-
neca, which they use in such quantities as often to injure their health
by producing spasms, etc.

"The third day is spent by the young men in hunting or fishing,
while the elder ones remain in the square and sleep, or continue
their black-drink, war-physic, etc., as they choose.   During the first
three days of busking, while the men are physicking, the women are
constantly bathing.   It is unlawful for any man to touch one of
them, even with the tip of his finger; and both sexes abstain rigidly
from all kinds of food or sustenance, and more particularly from salt.

"On the fourth day, the whole town are assembled in the square,
men, women, and children promiscuously, and devoted to convivi-
ality.   All the game killed the day before by the young hunters, is
given to the public; large quantities of new corn, and other provisions, are collected and cooked by the women over the new fire.
The whole body of the square is occupied with pots and pans of cooked
provisions, and they all partake in general festivity.   The evening
is spent in dancing, or other trifling amusements, and the ceremony
is concluded.

"N. B.—All the provisions that remain are a perquisite to the old
priest, or fire-maker.

"Anth^NY. Alex. M'Gillivray." [65]

---

[65] Schoolcraft, Ind. Tribes, vol. v, pp. 267-268.

In this ceremonial, as in the Kasihta busk recorded by Hawkins, the fire was kindled on the morning of the first day, but here the similarity ends. The women were shut out of the square on this first day, whereas it is evident they were not at Kasihta. The pasa was drunk on the second day instead of the first. It is to be noticed that this is the only town of the Creeks, so far as we know, in which the ási was sanctified along with the corn. I am inclined to think that this description leaves out a great deal, since no mention is made of the miko hoyanīdja or other medicines besides the pasa and ási, and because the bath with which the busk broke up is not recorded. The feasting day appears to have been at the end instead of the beginning.

The Apalachicola busk was held in the latter half of July, lasted only four days like the two preceding, and the days were named like those at Eufaula, the days of assembling, eating, fasting, and dispersing. About four people got together to decide on the war titles conferred at that time. One informant said they were taken from the names belonging to the clan of the aspirant's father, so that they changed every generation, but this was contradicted by everyone else. The people in the north bed selected some persons to call out the new names for the people in the west bed (the Chiefs' bed) who did not move from their places. Those who were to make the new fire were selected by the head men of the town from a certain clan and they held office for four years. This clan was probably the Bear. Certain men were also selected to place the four main sticks for the fire. The medicine was taken four times, just as the sun was on the eastern horizon, at noon, in the middle of the afternoon, and at sunset. Then they went to the river and dipped four times, facing the east. After that they could eat the new corn, beans, etc.

At Tuskegee, according to information obtained both by Doctor Speck and myself, there was a feast for the visitors from friendly towns on the first day, and during the same day the medicines were collected. On the second day the men fasted, the medicines were prepared and taken, the new fire lighted, a game of ball played, and finally the dancers bathed and danced all that night. The bath may, however, have occurred on the following morning (Silas Jefferson). The introduction of a ball game on this day seems unusual, as also another fact which I give on the authority of the last chief, that those who were going to fast rubbed their bodies with medicine and were scratched on the calves of the legs, the hips, and the hands up and down and crosswise, and also crosswise of their breasts. Two pots of hot medicine were taken first and then two pots of cold medicine later to induce vomiting.[66]

---

[66] The ball game and scarification seem to have been adopted from the Yuchi, who were neighbors of the Tuskegee after they moved west.

The Coweta busk has been given up for some time. As the capital town of the Lower Creeks, specific information regarding it would be of interest, but the notes I have are somewhat confusing and suggest that some of them apply to an earlier form of the busk and some to a later form. According to one informant, the day of gathering and the day of eating were identical. On the morning after this day six men went out very early before they had eaten anything and brought in the medicines. Those who were going to fast also abstained from food. The medicine was prepared and taken about noon. Afterwards there was a ball game between the men and women, followed by a dance which lasted until midnight. They rested from midnight until morning and next day began taking the medicine again. They took it four times a day for four days, fasted, and danced the feather dance and the gun dance. The night of the fourth day there was an all-night dance, and during this time the chief usually talked to them, warning them not to commit adultery or have sexual relations within the prescribed limits and bringing his remarks home by pointing to a long pole on which hung switches, and the ears, nose, and hair cut off of some earlier offender. Early next morning all went to the creek and dived into the water four times. Then they came back, all ate salted food, and the visitors, of whom there would then be crowds, were given food. That night they danced again, sometimes until midnight, sometimes all night. On the following morning the visitors prepared to go, and they gave a sign with the hand which signified "You friends that are here, now I am going." After the visitors had gone the chief made another speech to his own people, after which they, too, prepared to leave. The new fire was probably lighted on the first day of the fast, and four ears of corn were brought in and laid upon the sticks or beside them. Four fishes were also brought in. My informants did not know what was done with them, but, judging by the treatment accorded the meat at Tukabahchee, it may be considered probable that they were burned in the new fire. In late times there were only three men in the north bed during the fast, and these moved into the south bed when visitors were admitted. Women and children were admitted to seats in the east bed in later times, but anciently it was occupied by the younger men. There were two medicine pots, one of which contained both pasa and miko hoyanīdja and was warmed, while the other contained miko hoyanīdja alone and was cold.

According to a second informant the Coweta fasted one entire day and took what they called "the white nourishment" three days longer. This included all kinds of food but meat and salt. While this is probably correct I am doubtful whether we have here the original custom or a stage in the decay of the institution, a compromise to alleviate the asperity of the abstinence.

The account of this busk given by a third informant differs considerably and is probably the later form:

When the time was approaching for the annual busk the town chief and his assistants, who were all from thê same bed, would call together those Coweta men who lived near by and they would fix upon a date for the busk. Those Coweta living at a distance were notified in the usual way through a messenger who brought each a little bundle of sticks about as large as matches. One of these was thrown away every day until two were left, when the man knew that it was the day when he must start. On the day represented by the last stick all were gathered at the square ground. That night they had a dance, and in the morning before breakfast some persons were sent out after the different medicines. When these individuals came back they took a bath and then ate for the first time that day. The rest of the day all spent as suited them, and that night there was another dance. Next day was the day of feasting. If there were delegations of visitors from other towns of the same fire clan they would come in, one delegation at a time, the Chiaha, the Broken Arrows, etc. Each delegation would first dance around outside of the square toward the northeast while the Coweta men danced around toward the southwest. Then they came in and the visitors sat first in the north bed which had been vacated for them. As they did so they raised their right hands toward the Coweta (who were seated in the Chiefs' bed) but in a direction over the heads of the latter with a kind of sweep and said, "Are you friends here?" After remaining in the north bed a short time the visitors got up again and passed around in front of the Chiefs' bed. The Coweta chief would say "Have you come?" (àlahkitcka') and the chief of the visitors would answer "Yes" (Hehé). Each of the Coweta would then give a piece of tobacco to the visitor opposite him and the latter would give another piece in return. Then the visitors made the same salute as before and passed out to eat. After that 10 bowls of food were brought into the square all prepared. Then the visitors' women were called in and a bowl of food was sent to each delegation of visitors. The women took this to their own people and they feasted upon it.

Before this feast was served, however, the Coweta danced the gun dance (tabŏtckà obànga). Part of them came in with guns loaded only with powder and discharged them. Then all would run down to the creek while another squad armed with guns or bows and arrows pursued them all the way. All then bathed and returned. Women danced this dance and while they were doing so four men sang for them, using a drum and a cocoanut rattle. My informant added that nowadays this dance would be unsafe, for someone would certainly be shot to satisfy a grudge. After the women had been dismissed

with their bowls of food and the visitors had begun their feast the
Coweta commenced to fast, though they had in fact eaten nothing
that morning. They remained inside the bounds of the square and
could not so much as touch one of those who had eaten. In case a
man did so he was fined 25 or 50 cents. Each of the three medicines,
pasa, miko hoyanīdja, and ási, was mixed in a different vessel. The
bark of the miko hoyanīdja was scraped off before it was put into
the pot, but the pasa was put in whole, after which water was added,
the medicine man conjured it, and it was drunk hot. Two bearers
carried the medicines in long-handled gourds to those who were to
drink and uttered the yahola cry as they delivered it.[67] Each took
enough of it to make him vomit. All of the fasters took the medicine
four times during the day, but the day following was the regular
busk day. Early on the morning of that day before sunrise four
green logs about a yard long were brought in, placed in a cross shape,
each stick toward one of the cardinal points, and, by means of flint
and steel, fire was started at the place where all came together, the
sparks being caught upon some punk (totpáfka). There had been
a fire in this place during the preliminary days but before the new
fire was lighted all of the ashes from this were cleared away along
with all of those of the fire of the preceding year. In the time of my
informant this fire was not distributed to the camps. The sticks
were named after the points of the compass: South, wahála; north,
holīna; east, hasōsa ("rising sun"); and west, akálatka ("toward
the sunset"). Four roasting ears were brought in by persons who
had special charge of them, but my informant did not know what
was done with them. Two men called "the fishers" also went out
and brought in four fishes. Probably these were all burned in the
fire.

The medicine was taken at about 9, 12, 3, and 6 o'clock. After
the first medicine taking they danced the tcidahaia obánga, with the
usual feathered canes. One man led, accompanying himself with a
rattle, and the others responded. The song goes like this:

> hâtci dâ+hia
> hâtci dâ+hia
> hiha hī+hē+ + +

This refrain is repeated over and over many times. After this
was over the dancers went down to the creek to bathe. By this time
the four busk logs were about burned up and were all shoved on together and a big fire made up about which the people danced all
night. When the fast was over they partook of a meal in which
salt must be used. The dances on the last night were of various
kinds, and at intervals the chief made speeches to his people, telling
them how to behave, and in general inculcating virtues. Finally he

---

[67] This informant probably confused the customs connected with the ási with the usages regarding the
regular busk medicines.

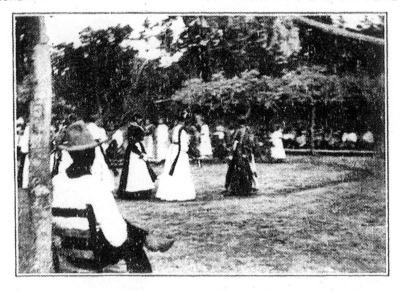

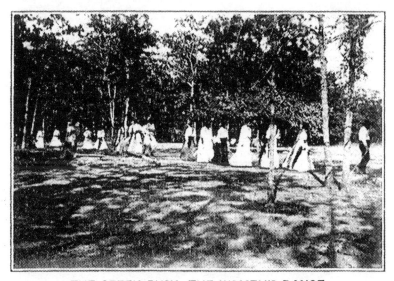

THE CREEK BUSK: THE WOMEN'S DANCE

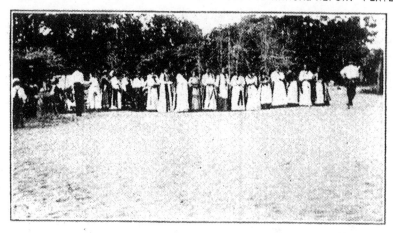

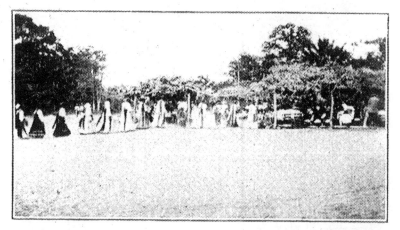

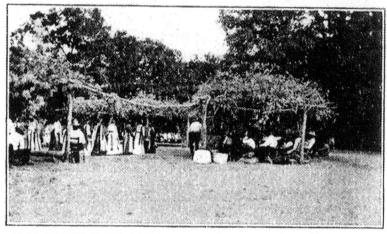

THE CREEK BUSK: WOMEN'S DANCE AT THE OKCHAI BUSK
IN 1912

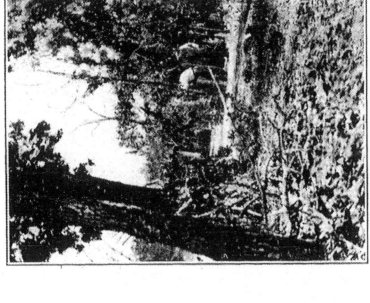

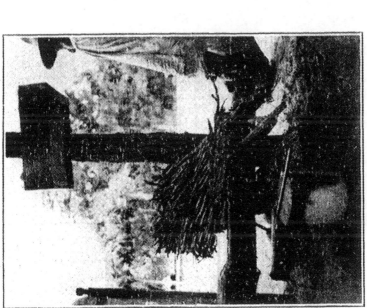

a. Box for tobacco, medicine, and drum in the Chiefs' Bed

b. Rite of the emetic

THE OKCHAI BUSK

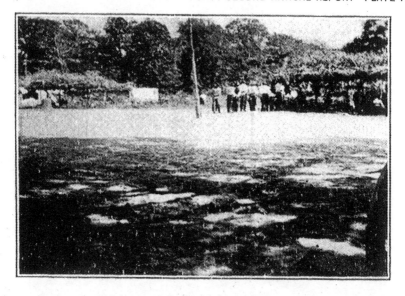

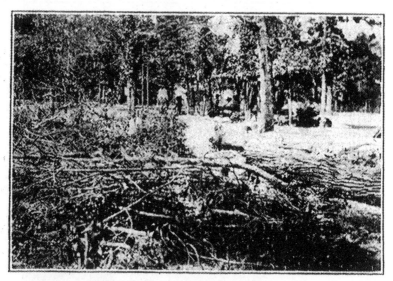

TAKING THE EMETIC AT OKCHAI

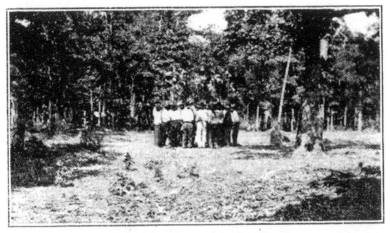

a. The tcitahaia or "feather dance"

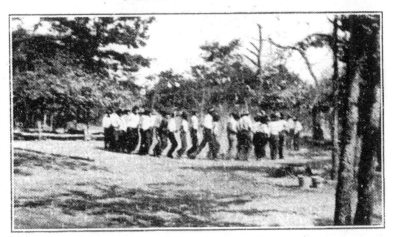

b. The tcitahaia or "feather dance"

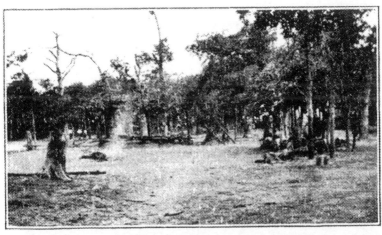

c. The Square Ground just after the fasters have left to bathe in a neighboring creek

THE CREEK BUSK

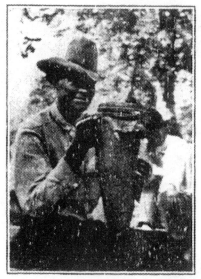

a. Drum

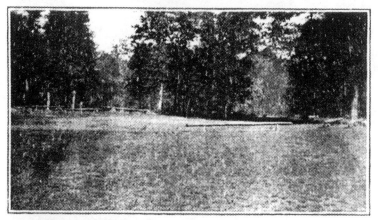

b. Ceremonial ground near Braggs, Okla., used by the Natchez, Creek, and Cherokee Indians

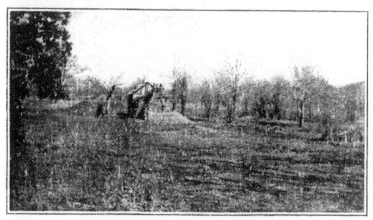

c. Home of the Kila or Prophet Yahola

THE CREEK AND NATCHEZ INDIANS

told them that if they lived through another year they must all assemble at the busk again. The next morning all went home. In commenting on the Coweta busk Bosomworth says that it was said to be an ancient custom for the chief to remain eight days in the square ground after the ceremony was over, a period which he spent "in performing several ceremonies and giving several necessary orders to his people." [68]

I find a conflicting note to the effect that the four busk logs were pushed in every day for four days, after which occurred the all night dance. Perhaps this applied to the older form of the busk. During this fast a man of the Aktayatci and two others were the only occupants of the north bed. Like one or two of the extant grounds, Coweta had a small house for the medicine pots.

I have myself witnessed the busks of Eufaula, Hilibi, and Okchai, all of which are similar (see pls. 8–12). At Eufaula the women's dance took place very late in the afternoon, at Hilibi it was very early, while at Okchai it was intermediate in time. The medicine at Okchai was taken considerably earlier in the day than at the two other places. The following additional notes were obtained from Tâl mutcási, the medicine maker of Asilanabi and Lâlogálga, who was familiar with the older customs.

When the ashes were removed from the old fire [69] by the warriors the camps were cleaned up and the warriors removed the ashes from them also. The women's medicine was placed southwest of the square, the men's medicine on the north end of the Chiefs' bed. The fire has been lighted in recent years with a match. Like the Tukabahchee they brought sand and laid it out in the place where the fire was to be lighted. Each of the four foundation sticks was conjured in advance and placed at the center of one of the four beds. A man was appointed to take charge of each stick and at a given word they approached the center and laid their four sticks down at the same instant in their proper positions.[69a] Anciently two sticks of post oak were used in making fire and later flint and steel were obtained from the French, and the sparks were caught upon true punk obtained from hickory or sycamore trees where the limbs have come away. When the punk caught fire, it was picked off, mixed with hay, and fanned until the whole burst into flames. The Asilanabi and Lâlogálga squares are within a few miles of each other, and nowadays (1912) they fast two days at Asilanabi and two days at Lâlogálga to make the four.

---

[68] The Bosomworth Journal Ms., S. C. Colls., p. 25.

[69] Burning coals were brought from the old square ground fire of the Okchai in Alabama by a leading man of the town and his heniha, kept alive during the migration west and buried about 2 feet under ground beneath the fire in the new square ground near Hanna, Okla. Ashes from the old Kasihta ground are also said to have been brought west for burial under the new ceremonial fire.

[69a] This treatment of the sticks is like that in the busk described by McGillivray. See p. 583.

Before the Civil War the Lutcapoga busk included a fast of four days, from which it may be inferred that the entire length was eight. This would apply as well to Tulsa, the mother town. This fast was from the evening of the first day to the morning after the fourth. Medicine was taken every day.

One description of the busk now remains to be considered—the one given by Adair. This is in several separate fragments which have to be pieced together, and there is, a running comparison with Hebrew customs which must be carefully excised. Of all accounts that have been preserved it is the most elaborate in detail, though the material is not systematically presented. Furthermore, we do not know certainly to which tribe or town it belongs. The context and the use of Chickasaw expressions throughout would lead us to suppose that we are having a Chickasaw ceremonial presented to us, but if so this is the only reference to a busk ceremonial in that tribe. As has been noted in several places, the Chickasaw were closely associated with the Creeks in many ways and had probably borrowed some of their customs—for a time there was a Chickasaw town among the Upper Creeks—but all other early writers are silent on the subject of a Chickasaw busk, and at the present day these Indians remember nothing whatever regarding such a ceremony. Their modern ceremonies are the Pishofa dances which differ from the Creek ceremonial in almost every particular. If this is a description of a Creek ceremony, it would probably be the busk of Coosa, Abihka, or Okfuskee, but this point along with the question whether it is Chickasaw or Creek must remain in doubt. In the square ground where it took place the Chiefs' bed was at the west, that of the Warriors at the south, that of the second men or henihàlgi north, and that of the Youths east. It is thus described:

"The Indians formerly observed the grand festival of the annual expiation of sin, at the beginning of the first new moon, in which their corn became fulleared; but for many years past they are regulated by the season of their harvest . . .

"As the first of the Neetak Hoollo, precedes a long strict fast of two nights and a day, they gormandize such a prodigious quantity of strong food, as to enable them to keep inviolate the succeeding fast, the sabbath of sabbaths, the Neetak Yah-ah: the feast lasts only from morning till sunset. Being great lovers of ripened fruits, and only tantalized as yet, with a near view of them; and having lived at this season, but meanly on the wild products of nature—such a fast as this may be truly said to afflict their souls, and to prove a sufficient trial of their religious principles. During the festival, some of their people are closely employed in putting their temple [the tcokofa] in proper order for the annual expiation; and others are painting the white cabbin, and the supposed holiest, with white clay; for it is a sacred, peaceable place, and white is the emblem. Some, at the same time are likewise painting the war-cabbin with red clay, or their emblematical red root, as occasion requires; while others of an inferior order, are covering all the seats of the beloved square with new mattresses, made out of fine splinters of long canes, tied together with flags. In the mean time, several of them are busy in sweeping the temple, clearing it of every supposed polluting thing, and carrying out the ashes from the hearth which perhaps had not been cleaned six times since the last year's general offering. Several towns join together to make the annual sacrifice; and, if the whole nation lies in a narrow compass, they make but one annual offering; by which means, either through a sensual or religious principle, they strike off the work with joyful hearts. Every thing being thus prepared, the Archi-magus [i. e. the medicine maker] orders some of his religious attendants to dig up the old hearth, or altar [in the center of the square], and to sweep out the remains that by chance might either be left, or drop down. Then he puts a few roots of the button-snake-root, with some green leaves of an uncommon small sort of tobacco, and a little of the new fruits, at the bottom of the fire-place, which he orders to be covered up with white marley clay, and wetted over with clean water.

"Immediately, the magi [the doctors] order them to make a thick arbour over the altar, with green branches of the various young trees, which the warriors had designedly chosen, and laid down on the outside of the supposed holy ground: the women, in the interim are busy at home in cleaning out their houses, renewing the old hearths, and cleaning all their culinary vessels, that they may be fit to receive the pretended holy fire, and the sanctified new fruits, according to the purity of the law; lest by a contrary conduct, they should incur damage in life, health, future crops, &c. It is fresh in the memory of the old traders, that formerly none of these numerous nations of Indians would eat, or even handle any part of the new harvest, till some of it had been offered up at the yearly festival by the Archi-magus, or those of his appointment, at their plantations, though the light harvest of the past year had forced them to give their women and children of the ripening fruits, to sustain life. Notwithstanding they are visibly degenerating, both in this, and every other religious observance, except what concerns war; yet their magi and old warriors live contentedly on such harsh food as nature affords them in the woods, rather than transgress that divine precept given to their forefathers.

"Having every thing in order for the sacred solemnity, the religious waiters carry off the remains of the feast, and lay them on the outside of the square; others of the inferior order carefully sweep out the smallest crumbs, for fear of polluting the first fruit offering; and before sunset, the temple must be cleared, even every kind of vessel or utensil, that had contained, or been used about any food in that expiring year. The women carry all off, but none of that sex, except half a dozen old beloved women are allowed in that interval to tread on the holy ground, till the fourth day. Now, one of the waiters proclaims with a loud voice, for all the warriors and beloved men, whom the purity of the law admits, to come and enter the beloved square, and observe the fast; he likewise exhorts all the women and children, and those who have not initiated themselves in war, to keep apart from them, according to law. Should any of them prove disobedient, the young ones would be dry-scratched, and the others stript of every thing they had on them . . .

"Their great beloved man, or Archi-magus, now places four sentinels [the dog-whippers], one at each corner of the holy square, to keep out every living creature as impure, except the religious order, and the warriors who are not known to have violated the law of the first-fruit-offering, and that of marriage, since the last year's expiation. Those sentinels are regularly relieved, and firm to their sacred trust; if they discerned a dog or cat on the out-limits of the holy square, before the first-fruit-offering was made, they would kill it with their arrows on the spot.

"They observe the fast till the rising of the second sun; and be they ever so hungry in that sacred interval the healthy warriors deem the duty so awful, and the violation so inexpressibly vicious, that no temptation would induce them to violate it; for, like the Hebrews, they fancy temporal evils are the necessary effect of their immoral conduct, and they would for ever ridicule and reproach the criminal for every bad occurrence that befel him in the new year, as the sinful author of his evils; and would sooner shoot themselves, than suffer such long-continued sharp disgrace. The religious attendants boil a sufficient quantity of button-snake-root, highly imbittered and give it round pretty warm, in order to vomit and purge their sinful bodies. Thus they continue to mortify and purify themselves, till the end of the fast . . .

"That the women and children, and those worthless fellows who have not hazarded their lives in defense of their holy places and things, and for the beloved people, may not be entirely godless, one of the old beloved men lays down a large quantity of the small-leafed tobacco, on the outside of a corner of the sacred square; and an old beloved woman carries it off, and distributes it to the sinners without, in large pieces, which they chew heartily, and swallow, in order to afflict their souls. She commends those who perform the duty with cheerfulness, and chides those who seem to do it unwillingly, by their wry faces on account of the bitterness of the supposed sanctifying herb. She distributes it in such quantities, as she thinks are equal to their capacity of sinning, giving to the reputed, worthless old He-hen-pickers, the proportion only of a child, because she thinks such spiritless pictures of men cannot sin with married women; as all the females love only the virtuous manly warrior, who has often successfully accompanied the beloved ark.

"In the time of this general fast, the women, children, and men of weak constitutions, are allowed to eat, as soon as they are certain the sun has begun to decline from his meridian altitude; but not before that period . . .

"The whole time of this fast may with truth be called a fast, and to the Archi-magus, to all the magi, and pretended prophets, in particular; for, by ancient custom, the former is obliged to eat of the sanctifying small-leafed tobacco, and drink the snake-root, in a separate hut for the space of three days and nights without any other subsistence, before the solemnity begins; besides his full portion along with the rest of the religious order, and the old war-chieftains, till the end of the general fast, which he pretends to observe with the strictest religion. After the first-fruits are sanctified, he lives most abstemiously till the end of the annual expiation only sucking water-melons now and then to quench thirst, and support life, spitting out the more substantial part . . . Thus the Indian religious are retentive of their sacred mysteries to death, and the Archi-magus is visibly thin and meagre at the end of the solemnity . . . The superannuated religious are also emulous in the highest degree, of excelling one another in their long fasting; for they firmly believe, that such an annual self-denying method is so highly virtuous, when joined to an obedience of the rest of their laws, as to be the infallible means of averting evil, and producing good things, through the new year. They declare that a steady virtue, through the divine co-operating favour, will infallibly insure them a lasting round of happiness.

"At the end of this solemn fast, the women by the voice of the crier, bring to the outside of the holy square, a plentiful variety of the old year's food newly dressed, which they lay down, and immediately return home; for every one of them know their several duties, with regard to both time and place. The centinels report the affair, and soon afterward the waiters by order go, and reaching their hands over the holy ground, they bring in the provisions, and set down before the famished multitude. Though most of the people may have seen them, they reckon it vicious and mean to shew a gladness for the end of their religious duties; and shameful to hasten the holy attendants, as they are all capable of their offices . . .

"Before noon, the temple is so cleared of every thing the women brought to the square, that the festival after that period, resembles a magical entertainment that had no reality in it, consisting only in a delusion of the senses. The women then carry the vessels from the temple to the water, and wash them clean for fear of pollution.

As soon as the sun is visibly declining from his meridian, this third day of the fast, the Archi-magus orders a religious attendant to cry aloud to the crowded town, that the holy fire is to be brought out for the sacred altar—commanding every one of them to stay within their own houses, as becomes the beloved people, without doing the least bad thing—and to be sure to extinguish, and throw away every spark of the old fire; otherwise, the devine fire will bite them severely with bad diseases, sickness, and a great many other evils, which he sententiously enumerates, and finishes his monitory caution, by laying life and death before them." [70]

The costume assumed by the Archi-magus or fire maker at this time is thus described by Adair:

"Before the Indian *Archi-magus* officiates in making the supposed holy fire, for the yearly atonement of sin, the Sagan clothes him with a white ephod, which is a waistcoat without sleeves. When he enters on that solemn duty, a beloved attendant spreads a white-drest buckskin on the white seat, which stands close to the supposed holiest, and then puts some white beads on it, that are given him by the people. Then the *Archi-magus* wraps around his shoulders a consecrated skin of the same sort, which reaching across under his arms, he ties behind his back, with two knots on the legs, in the form of a figure of eight. Another custom he observes on this solemn occasion, is, instead of going barefoot, he wears a new pair of buckskin white moccasenes made by himself, and stitched with the sinews of the same animal. The upper leather across the toes, he paints, for the space of three inches, with a few streaks of red—not with vermilion, for that is their continual war-emblem, but with a certain red root, its leaves and stalk resembling the ipecacuanha, which is their fixed red symbol of holy things. These shoes he never wears, but in the time of the supposed passover; for at the end of it, they are laid up in the beloved place, or holiest, where much of the like sort, quietly accompanies an heap of old, broken earthen ware, conchshells, and other consecrated things. . . . The American *Archi-magus* wears a breast-plate, made of a white conch-shell, with two holes bored in the middle of it, through which he puts the end of an otter-skin strap, and fastens a buckhorn white button to the outside of each . . . The Indian wears around his temples, either a wreath of swan-feathers, or a long piece of swan-skin doubled, so as only the fine snowy feathers appear on each side. And [he] wears on the crown of his head, a tuft of white feathers, which they call *Yatèra*. He likewise fastens a tuft of blunted wild Turkey cock-spurs, toward the toes of the upper part of his moccasenes. . . Thus appears the Indian Archi-magus . . . when he is to officiate in his pontifical function, at the annual expiation of sins. [71] . . .

---

[70] Adair, Hist. Am. Inds., pp. 100–105.   [71] Ibid., pp. 82–84.

"Now every thing is hushed. Nothing but silence all around: the Archi-magus, and his beloved waiter, rising up with a reverend carriage, steady countenance, and composed behaviour, go into the beloved place, or holiest, to bring them out the beloved fire. The former takes a piece of dry poplar, willow, or white oak, and having cut a hole, so as not to reach through it, he then sharpens another piece, and placing that with the hole between his knees, he drills it briskly for several minutes, till it begins to smoke—or, by rubbing two pieces together, for about a quarter of an hour, by friction he collects the hidden fire; which all of them reckon to immediately issue from the holy Spirit of fire . . . When the fire appears, the beloved waiter cherishes it with fine chips, or shaved splinters of pitch-pine, which had been deposited in the holiest: then he takes the unsullied wing of a swan, fans it gently, and cherishes it to a flame. On this, the Archi-magus brings it out in an old earthen vessel, whereon he had placed it, and lays it on the sacred altar, which is under an arbour, thick-weaved a-top with green boughs . . .

"Their hearts are enlivened with joy at the appearance of the reputed holy fire, as the divine fire is supposed to atone for all their past crimes, except murder: and the beloved waiter shews his pleasure, by his cheerful industry in feeding it with dry fresh wood; for they put no rotten wood on it . . . Although the people without, may well know what is transacting within, yet, by order, a crier informs them of the good tidings, and orders an old beloved woman to pull a basket-full of the new-ripened fruits, and bring them to the beloved square. As she before had been appointed, and religiously prepared for that solemn occasion, she readily obeys, and soon lays it down with a cheerful heart, at the out-corner of the beloved square. By ancient custom, she may either return home, or stand there, till the expiation of sin hath been made, which is thus performed—The Archi-magus, or fire-maker, rises from his white seat and walks northward three times round the holy fire, with a slow pace, and in a very sedate and grave manner, stopping now and then, and speaking certain old ceremonial words with a low voice and a rapidity of expression, which none understand but a few of the old beloved men, who equally secrete their religious mysteries, that they may not be prophaned. He then takes a little of each sort of the new harvest, which the old woman had brought to the extremity of the supposed holy ground, rubs some bear's oil over it, and offers it up together with some flesh, to the bountiful holy Spirit of fire as a first-fruit offering, and an annual oblation for sin. He likewise consecrates the button-snake-root, and the cusseena, by pouring a little of those two strong decoctions into the pretended holy fire. He then purifies the red and white seats with those bitter liquids, and sits down. Now, every one of the outlaws who had been catched a tripping, may safely creep out of their lurking holes, anoint themselves, and dress in their finest, to pay their grateful thanks at an awful distance, to the forgiving divine fire. A religious waiter is soon ordered to call to the women around, to come to the sacred fire: they gladly obey.—When they come to the outside of the quadrangular holy ground, the *Archi-magus* addresses the warriors, and gives them all the particular positive injunctions, and negative precepts they yet retain of the ancient law, relating to their own manly station. Then he changes his note, and uses a much sharper language to the women, as suspecting their former virtue. He first tells them very earnestly, that if there are any of them who have not extinguished the old evil fire, or have contracted any impurity, they must forthwith depart, lest the divine fire should spoil both them and the people; he charges them to be sure not to give the children a bad example of eating any unsanctified, or impure food, otherwise they will get full of worms, and be devoured by famine and diseases, and bring many other dangerous evils both upon themselves, and all the beloved, or holy people . . .

"In his female lecture, he is sharp and prolix; he urges them with much earnestness to an honest observance of the marriage-law, which may be readily executed, on account of the prevalent passion of self interest. Our own christian orators do not exert themselves with half the eloquence or eagerness, as when that is at stake which they most value. And the wary old savage has sense enough to know, that the Indian female virtue is very brittle, not being guarded so much by inward principle, as the fear of shame, and of incurring severe punishment; but if every bush of every thicket was an hundred-eyed Argos, it would not be a sufficient guard over a wanton heart. So that is natural they should speak much on this part of the subject, as they think they have much at stake. After that, he addresses himself to the whole body of the people, and tells them, in rapid bold language, with great energy, and expressive gestures of body, to look at the holy fire, which again has introduced all those shameful adulterous criminals into social privileges; he bids them not to be guilty of the like for time to come, but be sure to remember well, and strongly shake hands with the old beloved straight speech, otherwise the divine fire, which sees, hears, and knows them, will spoil them exceedingly, if at any time they relapse, and commit that detestable crime. Then he enumerates all the supposed lesser crimes, and moves the audience by the great motives of the hope of temporal good, and the fear of temporal evil, assuring them, that upon their careful observance of the ancient law, the holy fire will enable their prophets, the rain-makers, to procure them plentiful harvests, and give their war-leaders victory over their enemies—and by the communicative power of their holy things, health and prosperity are certain: but on failure, they are to expect a great many extraordinary calamities, such as hunger, uncommon diseases, a subjection to witchcraft, and captivity and death by the hands of the hateful enemy in the woods, where the wild fowls will eat the flesh, and beasts of prey destroy the remaining bones, so as they will not be gathered to their forefathers—because their ark abroad, and beloved things at home, would lose their virtual power of averting evil. He concludes, by advising them to a strict observance of their old rites and customs, and every thing shall go well with them. He soon orders some of the religious attendants to take a sufficient quantity of the supposed holy fire, and lay it down on the outside of the holy ground, for all the houses of the various associated towns, which sometimes lie several miles apart. The women, hating sharp and grave lessons, speedily take it up, gladly carry it home, and lay it down on their unpolluted hearths, with the prospect of future joy and peace." [72]

After these lectures the women hasten to prepare food of the new year on the new fire which they have obtained, and meanwhile a dance takes place which is described in a different place by Adair as follows:

"While their sanctified new fruits are dressing, a religious attendant is ordered to call six of their old beloved women to come to the temple, and dance the beloved dance with joyful hearts, according to the old beloved speech. They cheerfully obey, and enter the supposed holy ground in solemn procession, each carrying in her hand a bundle of small branches of various green trees; and they join the same number of old magi, or priests, who carry a cane in one hand adorned with white feathers, having likewise green boughs in their other hand, which they pulled from their holy arbour, and carefully place there, encircling it with several rounds. Those beloved men have their heads dressed with white plumes; but the women are decked in their finest, and anointed with bear's-grease, having small tortoise shells, and white pebbles [or beads], fastened to a piece of white-drest deerskin, which is tied to each of their legs [on the outside].

"The eldest of the priests leads the sacred dance, a-head of the innermost row, which of course is next to the holy fire. He begins the dance round the supposed holy fire, by invoking Yah, after their usual manner, on a bass key, and with a short accent; then he sings Yo Yo, which is repeated by the rest of the religious procession; and he continues his sacred invocations and praises, repeating the divine word, or notes, till they return to the same point of the circular course, where they began: then He He in like manner, and Wah Wah. While dancing they never fail to repeat those notes; then *Heleluiah*, *Halelu-Yah*, and Aleluiah and Alelu-Yah, 'Irradia-

[72] Adair, Hist. Am. Inds., pp. 105-108.

tion to the divine essence,' with great earnestness and fervor, till they encircle the altar, while each strikes the ground with right and left feet alternately, very quick, but well-timed. Then the awful drums join the sacred choir, which incite the old female singers to chant forth their pious notes, and grateful praises before the divine essence, and to redouble their former quick joyful steps, in imitation of the leader of the sacred dance, and the religious men a-head of them. What with the manly strong notes of the one, and the shrill voices of the other, in concert with the bead-shells, and the two sounding, drum-like earthen vessels, with the voices of the musicians who beat them, the reputed holy ground echoes with the praises of Yo He Wah . . . They continue their grateful divine hymns for fifteen minutes, when the dance breaks up." [73]

At the same time the ási was being prepared. Adair continues:

"The Archi-magus sends a religious attendant to pull some cusseena, or yopon, belonging to the temple; and having parched it brown on the altar, he boils it with clear running water in a large earthen pot, about half full; it has such a stong body, as to froth above the top by pouring it up and down with their consecrated vessels, which are kept only for that use: of this they drink now and then, till the end of the festival, and on every other religious occasion from year to year. Some of the old beloved men, through a religious emulation in sanctifying themselves, often drink this, and other bitter decoctions, to such excess, as to purge themselves very severely,— when they drink it, they always invoke Yo He Wah [i. e., always utter the yahola cry].

"If any of the warriors are confined at home by sickness, or wounds, and are either deemed incapable or unfit to come to the annual expiation, they are allowed one of the consecrated conch-shells-full of their sanctifying bitter cusseena, by their magi. The traders hear them often dispute for it, as their proper due, by ancient custom: and they often repeat their old religious ceremonies to one another, especially that part which they imagine most affects their present welfare; the aged are sent to instruct the young ones in these particulars . . .

"Though the Indians do not eat salt in their first-fruit oblation till the fourth day; it is not to be doubted but they formerly did. They reckon they cannot observe the annual expiation of sins, without bear's oil, both to mix with that yearly offering, and to eat with the new sanctified fruits; and some years they have a great deal of trouble in killing a sufficient quantity of bears for the use of this religious solemnity, and their other sacred rites for the approaching year; for at such seasons they are hard to be found, and quite lean. The traders commonly supply themselves with plenty of this oil from winter

---

[73] Adair, Hist. Am. Inds., pp. 96-98.

to winter; but the Indians are so prepossessed with a notion of the white people being all impure and accursed, that they deem their oil as polluting on those sacred occasions, as Josephus tells us the Jews reckoned that of the Greeks. An Indian warrior will not light his pipe at a white man's fire if he suspects any unsanctified food has been dressed at it in the new year. And in the time of the new-ripened fruits, their religious men carry a flint, punk, and steel, when they visit us, for fear of polluting themselves by lighting their pipes at our supposed Loak ookproose [Luak okpulosi], 'accursed fire,' and spoiling the power of their holy things. The polluted would, if known, be infallibly anathamatized, and expelled from the temple, with the women, who are suspected of gratifying their vicious taste. During the eight days festival, they are forbidden even to touch the skin of a female child; if they are detected, either in cohabiting with, or laying their hand on any of their own wives, in that sacred interval, they are stripped naked, and the offender is universally deemed so atrocious a criminal, that he lives afterwards a miserable life. Some have shot themselves dead, rather than stand the shame, and the long year's continual reproaches cast upon them, for every mischance that befalls any of their people, or the ensuing harvest,—a necessary effect of the divine anger, they say, for such a crying sin of pollution. An instance of this kind I heard happened some years ago in Talase, a town of the Muskohge, seven miles above the Alebama garrison.[73a]

"[The food having been prepared] the women now with the utmost cheerfulness, bring to the outside of the sacred square, a plentiful variety of all those good things, with which the divine fire has blessed them in the new year; and the religious attendants lay it before them, according to their stated order and reputed merit. Every seat is served in a gradual succession, from the white and red imperial long broad seats, and the whole square is soon covered: frequently they have a change of courses of fifty or sixty different sorts, and thus they continue to regulate themselves, till the end of the festival; for they reckon they are now to feast themselves with joy and gladness, as the divine fire is appeased for past crimes, and has propitiously sanctified their weighty harvest.[74] . . .

"When we consider how sparingly they eat in their usual way of living, it is surprising to see what a vast quantity of food they consume on their festival days. It would equally surprise a stranger to see how exceedingly they vary their dishes, their dainties consisting only of dried flesh, fish, oil, corn, beans, pease, pompions, and wild fruit. During this rejoicing time, the warriors are dresst in their wild martial array, with their heads covered with white down; they carry feathers of the same colour, either in their hands, or fastened

[73a] Adair, Hist. Am. Inds., pp. 108-109.   [74] Ibid., pp. 98-99.

to white scraped canes, as emblems of purity, and scepters of power, while they are dancing in three circles, and singing their religious praises around the sacred arbour, in which stands the holy fire. Their music consists of two clay-pot drums, covered on the top with thin wet deer-skins, drawn very tight, on which each of the noisy musicians beats with a stick, accompanying the noise with their voices; at the same time, the dancers prance it away, with wild and quick sliding steps, and variegated postures of the body, to keep time with the drums, and the rattling calabashes shaked by some of their religious heroes, each of them singing their old religious songs, and striking notes in tympano et choro. Such is the graceful dancing, as well as the vocal and instrumental music of the red Hebrews on religious and martial occasions, which they must have derived from early antiquity. Toward the conclusion of the great festival, they paint and dress themselves anew, and give themselves the most terrible appearance they possibly can. They take up their war-instruments, and fight a mock-battle in a very exact manner: after which, the women are called to join in a grand dance, and if they disobey the invitation they are fined. But as they are extremely fond of such religious exercise, and deem it productive of temporal good, all soon appear in their finest apparel, as before suggested, decorated with silver ear-bobs, or pendants to their ears, several rounds of white beads about their necks, rings upon their fingers, large wire or broad plates of silver on their wrists, their heads shining with oil, and torrepine-shells containing pebbles, fastened to deer-skins, tied to the outside of their legs. Thus adorned, they join the men in three circles, and dance a considerable while around the sacred fire, and then they separate.

"At the conclusion of this long and solemn festival, the Archi-magus orders one of the religious men to proclaim to all the people, that their sacred annual solemnity is now ended, and every kind of evil averted from the beloved people, according to the old straight beloved speech; they must therefore paint themselves, and come along with him according to ancient customs. As they know the stated time, the joyful sound presently reaches their longing ears: immediately they fly about to grapple up a kind of chalky clay, to paint themselves white. By their religious emulation, they soon appear covered with that emblem of purity, and join at the outside of the holy ground, with all who had sanctified themselves within it, who are likewise painted, some with streaks, and others all over, as white as the clay can make them: recusants would undergo a heavy penalty. They go along in a very orderly solemn procession, to purify themselves in running water. The Archi-magus heads the bold train— his waiter next—the beloved men according to their seniority—and the warriors by their reputed merit. The women follow them in the same orderly manner, with all the children that can walk, behind them, ranged commonly according to their height; the very little ones they carry in their arms. Those, who are known to have eaten of the unsanctified fruits, bring up the rear. In this manner the procession moves along, singing . . . till they get to the water, which is generally contiguous, when the Archi-magus jumps into it, and all the holy train follow him, in the same order they observed from the temple. Having purified themselves, or washed away their sins, they come out with joyful hearts, believing themselves out of the reach of temporal evil, for their past vicious conduct; and they return in the same religious cheerful manner, into the middle of the holy ground, where having made a few circles, singing and dancing around the altar, they thus finish their great annual festival, and depart in joy and peace.[75]

In a note he adds:

"They are so strictly prohibited from eating salt, or flesh-meat, till the fourth day, that during the interval, the very touch of either is accounted a great pollution: after that period, they are deemed lawful to be eaten. All the hunters, and able-bodied men, kill and barbecue wild game in the woods, at least ten days before this great festival, and religiously keep it for their sacred use." [76]

If this was indeed a Chickasaw ceremony it declined rapidly, and the declension had begun even in Adair's time, for he says: "As they degenerate, they lengthen their dances, and shorten the time of their fasts and purifications; insomuch, that they have so exceedingly corrupted their primitive rites and customs, within the space of the last thirty years, that, at the same rate of declension, there will not be long a possibility of tracing their origin, but by their dialects, and war-customs." [76] It may be added that a comparison of the earlier and later forms of the busk tends to bear out Adair's statement with reference to the lengthening of the dances and the shortening of the fasts and purifications. In other words, the social features progressively expanded at the expense of those of a strictly religious nature. It is a process common in all parts of the world where faith in an institution is gradually decaying. In this case the decay was due not so much to the direct influence of European missionaries as to the general modifying tendencies accompanying the advance of white civilization.

A word or two might be added regarding the busk of the Alabama Indians now living in Texas. It is rather curious to find that the Alabama in Oklahoma who have been in close contact with the whites still maintain a busk ground, while those in Texas, though they are

[75] Adair, Hist. Am. Inds., pp. 108–111.   [76] Ibid., p. 98.

comparatively remote from white settlements of any size, gave theirs up so long ago that only the oldest people know much about it. The Alabama kept their busk some time in June. It was thought that after it was held the corn would not hurt anybody but before that it was wrong to touch it. If anyone did not take part in the ceremony the other people would not talk to him, let him come into their houses, or have anything to do with him. They said "it was wrong." At the beginning of this ceremony each family brought a quantity of ears of corn already roasted to the square ground and it was put up on a scaffolding made of canes and raised on forked posts to a height of perhaps 4 feet. Then all the people came there and danced until midnight. At about that time some of the roasting ears were shelled and a few men took a handful apiece and threw it over the house. This was done four times. What was left they ate. Then one man blew through a cane into a pot of medicine which had previously been heated and all had to drink some of this. After drinking it they went away and vomited it up. They used the pasa (Koasati pasé), but there was another medicine in the pot with it. The taking of this medicine was thought to bring good luck and health. Early on the following morning the new fire was made in the square by twirling a stick from a bush called hàsa'làpo against a stick of slippery elm (bàkca). Previously all of the fires in the village had been extinguished, and each woman carried home some of the new fire. The new fire is said to have been made out in the woods and was brought into the square from there. Next day the people went home and roasted more corn which they brought to the same place. In the evening they danced, threw more corn over the roof, and again ate. They did this four nights in succession and then the ceremony ended.

The "old dance" was probably danced at this time, but I am not sure. As the Alabama performed it there was one drummer and he had one assistant to help him sing. There were five or six songs. The dancers went about the fire in two files, the women next to the fire, the men outside. Each dancer held his hands clasped in front and twisted his body from side to side as he proceeded. They danced around the fire once, stopping and completing the first song at the same time. Then they went around singing another song and stopped again at the end of one circuit. When the last song was taken up they went around twice before they stopped.

Ceremonies modeled after those of the Creek busk seem to have spread to the Cherokee within recent years, though certain changes have been introduced. When I first visited the few surviving speakers of Natchez near Braggs, Okla., the ceremonial ground of the Indians near by had the four cabins typical of Creek practice and was resorted to by Natchez, Creeks, and Cherokee,[77] but on my next

<hr/>

[77] See Bull. 43, Bur. Amer. Ethn., Pl. 10.

visit the ground had been moved and seven cabins had been substituted for the four (pl. 13, *b*). This was to conform to the sacred seven of the Cherokee and the seven clan system, each cabin being occupied by some one of the seven clans. Afterwards I visited two or three other ceremonial grounds in the Cherokee Nation, all with the same arrangment, but I know practically nothing regarding the ceremonies which take place there. My Natchez informant stated that anciently the miko used to stand in front of the fire in the ceremonial ground holding the peace pipe with the stem away from him and the other men would then come in succession, take it from his hands and puff four times toward the sky in the direction of the deity. This happened just before they began dancing. He also stated that they had about three special "stomp dances" during the year, accompanied by feasting and a ball game, from which it appears either that he is citing the Creek custom or that the Natchez usage was the same.

We will now give an abstract of the more important ceremonials which have been described:

THE CHIAHA BUSK (ELLIS CHILDERS)

First day.—Camping day, when the people go into camp about the square ground.

Second day.—Visitors' day, when visitors from towns of the same fire clan are entertained.

Third day.—Feasting day; visitors and townspeople both eat quantities of food.

Fourth day.—Visitors leave for their homes early in the morning. The men of the town fast.

Fifth day.—Fines are collected from those who failed to attend and the proceeds, being usually in the form of eatables, are consumed along with other food.

THE KASIHTA BUSK (HAWKINS)

First day.—Square cleaned. Asi or black drink is brewed. The new fire made. The turkey dance performed by women of the Turkey clan. Pasa prepared and drunk. The tadpole dance performed. They dance the heniha dance all night.

Second day.—Women dance the itcha dance (not the "gun dance" as Hawkins says). Shortly after noon the men bathe in the river. They feast on new corn.

Third day.—The men sit in the square.

Fourth day.—The women get and carry home the new fire. The first four logs are entirely consumed on this day. The fasters eat salt. They dance the long dance.

Fifth day.—Four new logs are procured for the fire. Asi is drunk.

Sixth day.—The men remain in the square.

Seventh day.—The men remain in the square.

Eighth day.—Old man's tobacco (hitci pàkpàgi) is thrown into the fire. The fasters anoint themselves with clay and ashes and go to the river with much ceremony to bathe.

THE EUFAULA BUSK (JACKSON LEWIS)

First day.—Day of assembling.

Second day.—Women's dance is held during the day. A general dance all night.

Third day.—The new fire is kindled. Medicines are dug, prepared, and taken four times. Between drinkings speeches are delivered and names given out. They dance the tcitahaia dance. A general dance follows lasting all night.

Fourth day.—Day when the busk breaks up.

THE OTCIAPOFA BUSK (SWAN)

First day.—New fire is made. Four ears of corn are placed upon it. Asi is prepared, some poured into the fire, and the rest drunk. The new fire is distributed.

Second day.—The men take the pasa.

Third day.—The younger men go hunting and fishing; the elders stay in the square and take àsi.

Fourth day.—There is a feast and dance this evening.

THE COWETA BUSK (FIRST INFORMANT)

First day.—Day of assembling and eating.

Second day.—The new fire is lighted and corn and fish burned in it. Medicines are prepared and taken about noon. They dance the tcitahaia dance and the gun dance. There is a ball game. A general dance until midnight.

Third day.—Medicines are taken again four times; they dance the tcitahaia and gun dances.

Fourth day.—The same.

Fifth day.—The same. That night the chief delivers speeches and they dance until morning.

Sixth day.—All bathe in the creek. They eat food that has been salted and serve their visitors.

Seventh day.—The visitors leave. The town chief makes a speech to his own people, who then leave for home.

THE COWETA BUSK (SECOND INFORMANT) [77a]

First day.—All assemble at the square. They dance all night.

Second day.—The medicines are gathered. They dance all night.

[77a] This is the "third informant" cited on page 587.

Third day.—The day of feasting; visitors are entertained. The Coweta Indians fast and take medicines four times. The Coweta Indians dance the gun dance. They bathe in the creek.

Fourth day.—The fast day proper. The old fireplace is cleaned up and the new fire lighted. Four ears of corn and four fishes are brought to the place and burned. They take medicines four times; after the first time they dance the tcitahaia dance. They eat salted food. The chief makes speeches to them in the evening and they dance all night.

Fifth day.—All go home.

<h3 style="text-align:center">THE TUKABAHCHEE BUSK</h3>

First day.—All assemble.

Second day.—The women dance. Materials for the new fire and medicines are procured. They dance at night. The men sleep in the square.

Third day.—The men fast. Ashes are cleared from the old fireplaces, sand spread there, the new fire lighted, four ears of corn put into the fire and the fire distributed. Medicines are prepared and taken; some youths get the stomp dance medicines and take their busk medicines after they come back. All go to dive into the creek. They break their fast. There is an all-night dance.

Fourth day.—All rest; later some play ball. There is a feast on green corn and other vegetable foods. A council is held in the evening and directions sent out for a hunt on the following day. An all-night dance follows.

Fifth day.—The men go hunting.

Sixth day.—A piece of beef is brought and put into the fire. A war dance is held. A feast follows, consisting largely of meat; salt is used.

Seventh day.—There is a second fast.

Eighth day.—The chief delivers an address to his people and dismisses them for the year.

<h3 style="text-align:center">THE TUKABAHCHEE BUSK (OLDER FORM)</h3>

The first two days are the same.

Third day.—Ashes are cleared from the old fireplaces, and sand spread there for fires and to rest the copper shields upon. The shields are washed in the creek and placed on the sand. The fire is lighted, four ears of corn are burned in it, and it is distributed. Asi is prepared and given to the shield bearers. The bearers dance with the shields. Pretended scouts go out and on coming back are given tobacco. There is a stomp dance that night to which no women are admitted.

Fourth day.—A gun dance is held, including a mock fight. All bathe in the creek. They rest the remainder of the day. The dumpling dance is sometimes indulged in in the evening.

Fifth day.—The men go hunting.

Sixth day.—A piece of meat is put into the fire. They bathe in the creek and the "busk is destroyed." The women dance. The old dance is danced. Necessary work is done.

Seventh day.—They fast all day. At night there is a stomp dance.

Eighth day.—The chief delivers a lecture to the people and they go home.

THE BUSK DESCRIBED BY ADAIR

First day.—The square is thoroughly cleaned and painted; new coverings are made for the seats; the fireplace is cleaned out. A feast follows, the remains of which are afterwards carefully removed. The men are called into the square in the evening to fast.

Second day.—The men fast all day. The medicines are taken. Women, children, and men in feeble health fast until noon and then eat.

Third day.—Food is brought by the women to the edge of the square where it is taken by the men and eaten, the feast being completed before noon. All of the fires are extinguished, and a new fire is made in the tcokofa. New corn, bear's oil, the pasa, and the àsi are put into the fire. The medicine maker ("archi-magus") lectures the people. The women get the new fire and take it home. Six old women dance in the tcokofa. (The àsi has been prepared while the above was going on and is taken from time to time.)

Fourth day.—The women prepare a great feast. A mock battle is fought. A big dance takes place. All plunge into running water.

Adair is somewhat confusing, inasmuch as he speaks of the ceremony sometimes as lasting four days, sometimes eight.[78] In the enumeration of the eight, the three or four days in which the medicine maker had to fast in preparation may be included. Accounts of the other ceremonies are too fragmentary to be analyzed; the value of the material they contain is principally as illustrative of the rest.

With the preceding may be compared the Yuchi ceremonial as recorded by Doctor Speck. He has begun numbering the days of this ceremony with that which we have called the "day of feasting," making seven in all, but before this is a day of assembling which, if added to the rest, makes the conventional eight. In order to compare this ceremonial more satisfactorily with the others, I shall venture to change the numbering by reckoning the day of assembling as the first.

First day.—The people assemble.

---

[78] Adair, Hist. Am. Inds., p. 109.

Second day.—Materials for the new fire and the medicines are procured. A sumptuous evening meal is served. In the evening the big turtle dance takes place. The town chief delivers a speech.

Third day.—The medicine plants are brought to the square. The new fire is lighted. The medicines are prepared. The males of the town are scratched. The medicines are taken. The men go to the creek, wash off their paint, and cleanse their hands, the town chief remaining meanwhile in the square. Some ears of corn are rubbed over the bathers and some are thrown into the fire. The men in the square smoke tobacco. The town chief makes a short speech. Food is brought into the square and eaten, the fast being ended. The fasters retire to their camps to rest. The young boys have a ball game. The young men play ball. They dance all night in the square. (The feather dance is sometimes danced once before and once after taking the medicines; the gun dance was performed in the day by one town and in the evening by another.)

Fourth day.—The assembly temporarily disbands, most of the people going to their own homes.

Fifth day.—The people remain at home.

Sixth day.—The people reassemble at the square.

Seventh day.—A feast consisting of meat takes place at noon. At night there is a general dance.

Eighth day.—The ceremonial gathering breaks up.

The fourth or fifth day, perhaps both the fourth and the fifth, undoubtedly corresponded to the day spent in hunting mentioned in describing some of the Creek busks. In later times they merely went to the store instead of to the forest.

Some additional remarks may now be made regarding certain features of these busks. First we will take up the medicines. Anciently it is probable that four pots of medicine were used but now the number is reduced to two. The àsi was brewed by itself and seems to have been used at a different time during the ceremonies from that in which the pasa and the miko hoyanīdja were taken. One of the chief reasons for giving up àsi was the fact that the plant was not readily obtainable in the western homes of the Creeks. The pasa was usually in a pot by itself and it was warmed over a slow fire; in Chiaha the miko hoyanīdja was combined with several other medicines, among which were the ice weed (hitūtàbi) and cedar, and taken cold. At Tukabahchee hitci pàkpàgi is used as a "foundation" for the warm medicine or adiloga, and the pasa was put with these, while the miko hoyanīdja was taken cold. The 10 medicines composing the adilō′ga were spiceweed, cedar, strawberry, grapevine, blackberry, mistletoe, horsemint, maremint, everlasting, and a forked oak limb, one of the arms of which while still on the tree had pointed toward the west and the other toward the south. Sometimes they added more medicines, as for instance the dewberry, and for

each one they made a mark on the ground. At Eufaula they formerly
used the pasa and miko hoyanīdja, but now have given up the pasa.
The wormseed, taken just before the busk broke off, was considered
a vermifuge. At Kasihta, according to Hawkins, the pasa, which the
early writers call "the war physic," was drunk on the afternoon of
the first day, while the miko hoyanīdja, and thirteen other medicine
plants were put into two pots and taken on the last day.[79] The
two bearers of the medicine in that town in later times belonged to the
Alligator clan. At Tuskegee two pots of hot medicine were taken,
followed by two pots of cold medicine. At Coweta the pasa, miko
hoyanīdja, and àsi were each mixed in a separate pot. At the Fish
Pond town on the morning after the men had finished drinking two
men carried medicine to the women for their households. What was
left was poured out around the fire. It was thought that the fire
would become too hot if the medicine was poured upon it, probably
from the magic qualities communicated. On the other hand a Hilibi
man said that a little medicine was put on the fire by his own people
and the Eufaula Indians to subdue it and in this way reduce the
likelihood of fevers during the ensuing year.[80] Anciently the medicine was not poured out in this way, though the custom has been in
vogue for some time. At Nuyaka the old fire was put out by two men,
one of the Bear and one of the Wind clan, who walked around it four
times and then threw medicine on it, after which it was rebuilt and
the busk went on. The Mikasuki used pasa, miko hoyanīdja (Mikasuki ayikstànage), adilōga, and àsi (Mikasuki àsoktce'), but when
their square ground in Florida was destroyed by the whites and
Coweta they gave up the last.

The following information was vouchsafed by an old Hilibi Indian
during the busk at Eufaula:

When the medicine maker blows into the medicine all of the men
in the beds are very quiet and attentive and are absorbed in what
is going on. When he blows, the god that is in him goes into the
medicine from the soul of the blower. He always blows facing the
east so as to see the rising sun over the fire, for the fire was thought
to be an important and useful thing which the Indians did not create
but which was given them by God, and it was reverenced accordingly. The miko hoyanīdja is taken to ward off ills, to act as a
kind of wall about the people against pestilence or any kind of
disease. The mashed medicine should be taken home after the
busk and used in cases of sickness. The pasa is "for the coldness of
the corn." It is thought to be especially for the children and is
put on the heads and hands of women, children, and men. Properly
it is not a medicine but a thank offering for the corn of the preceding
year.

[79] See pp. 577–578.   [80] See also Adair's description, p. 595.

The new fire at Eufaula is now lighted with a match, but earlier flint and steel were used and still earlier two sticks of wood. Jackson Lewis said that the lower stick was taken from a tree called afoslibakfa which looks something like a pawpaw and the bark of which may be stripped up from the root very readily (wahu tree—Loughridge). The twirling stick was a piece of cane. Six or seven men took turns at this and sometimes Jackson Lewis affirmed that a bow was used. The fire is now carried down to the camps but not to the homes. Pope, whose acquaintance was particularly with Broken Arrow, says that the base stick was a dry piece of poplar and the twirling stick a stick of sassafras, and that the fire making was done by the medicine maker.[81] This appears to have been the usual ancient custom. Bartram mentions the addition of resin as an aid in fire production.[82] Jackson Knight, who belonged to the western Abihka town, affirmed that the four foundation sticks were intended to point to the entries, as was also the case with the Tukabahchee sticks.

The busk dances may be summarized as follows:

Itcha obànga,[83] *called in Eufaula ni'ta obànga (the daylight dance).*— This is the women's dance which took place on the day just before the fast day proper. The atasa and attachments carried by the leading women seem to indicate that this was originally a scalp or war dance, and this view is strengthened by the fact that at Nuyaka the management of it was in the hands of the occupants of the south bed, all of whom belonged to Tciloki or war clans. On the other hand, at Eufaula it was conducted by the White clans.

Tcitahaia, popularly known as the "feather dance" because the dancers have canes in their hands with feathers fastened at the ends.— This is distinctly a peace dance. At Tukabahchee the feathers were attached to the canes by members of the Bird clan, and in some towns they were feathers of the little white heron (fus hàtka) or the white crane. In Tukabahchee only the White clans carried feathers of this kind, the Tciloki carrying eagle feathers. The song accompanying it is said to have been obtained by a certain man from the summer crane. He was traveling along in a certain place, heard this song, and wondered for a long time what caused it, but finally discovered that it was a crane. The entire dance was also under the supervision of the White clans, and nowadays it is said that the feathers and the dance both typify the peace with the American Government, while the clearing out of the white yard signifies that they are true to the obligations of that treaty. I was told that when the Tukabahchee danced the feather dance, which they no longer do, when they took up their feathered canes, they rubbed out the prints made by the butt ends of the wands with the soles of their feet.

---

[81] Pope, Tour, p. 55.

[82] Bartram, Trans. Am. Eth Soc., vol. III, p. 27.

[83] This word is confounded by Hawkins with Itca'. "gun." See p. 578.

Obànga tcàpko, "the long dance."—This was danced in the evening. At Tukabahchee it was danced on the evening of the third day, the dancers carrying feathered wands as in the feather dance, and it was also danced on the afternoon of that day, the dancers holding the shields. It is not now much used.

Tabotcka obànga, "the gun dance."—This was usually danced early in the morning after the fast day and took place on the ball ground. In this dance firearms were discharged, and human effigies were made and shot at. Sometimes they painted these with pokeberry juice, made them look as if they had been wounded or killed, and carried them out in that condition. The presentation was frequently so realistic that the uninitiated were very much frightened.

Obànga atcūli, "the old dance."—This was danced on the evening of the fast day after the fast was over and marked the time when the fasters were perfectly free. It was, however, danced only by the men, who at that time wore tortoise-shell rattles on their legs.

Obànga hadjo, "the drunken dance."—This was danced on the night after the preceding and usually when the concourse was ready to break up.

Paìhka obànga, "the war dance."—This was danced at the time of the first stomp dance of the season at Tukabahchee by a man named itci yàhola.[83a]

The dumpling dance was sometimes danced for amusement at Tukabahchee on the evening of the fourth day.

Anciently Hawkins tells us that the turkey dance was performed by women of the Turkey clan on the first day of the busk and later on the same day came the tadpole and henìha dances, the latter at night.[84]

Many other dances, especially the animal dances, were introduced on the last night. They began then with the common or stomp dance (sătkita obànga) which lasted until about midnight, after which the animal dances were introduced and continued until morning.

Speeches were usually made by the chief's yatika, but the war speaker (holibonaia) might be called upon on occasions of national emergency and if any good speaker was known to be present among the visitors he would be invited to address the assemblage. According to one man a tàstànàgi was chosen to make a speech several times during the night of the general dance, and according to another speeches were made by men of the Tcilokis, but it was the general opinion that the yatika was chosen from any clan. Before he spoke a man would spit four times very deliberately to each side and repeat a formula. Formal speeches usually began with the word Ta-a-a intukà'stci, "Now everybody's attention."

[83a] See p. 557. [84] See pp. 577–578.

These speeches were couched in a particular form, contained certain peculiar words, and were uttered in a rhythmic manner which may be likened to the intoning of a religious service. The late Chief G. W. Grayson, of Eufaula, Okla., supplied a short speech after the ancient type which is incorporated herewith. Such a speech was known as the "long talk" and it was delivered by the chief's yatika or "long talker" just before the women danced the Itcha obánga or "daylight dance."[84a] Mr. Grayson says: "You will notice the speaker often ends his sentences with 'he says so,' because the chief never makes a public address. You will understand that this is not a stereotyped copy of a talk that would in every instance be delivered at such a gathering, but *about* such as I have often heard, only this is abbreviated, as it fails to touch upon many subjects usually included in such talks. . . As I have told you, if this style of public speaking was ever the only way the Creeks spoke, it is now long since obsolete, except at the 'busks' and just before entering the ball play." Mr Grayson has kindly furnished both a line for line and a free translation of this speech, the original being in the official Creek orthography. [84b]

TEXT WITH INTERLINEAR TRANSLATION

Ta intukvstsi!
1. Hayomate:
   Now:
2. Momet umvres en kuhmit?
   Thus it shall be I thought for them,
3. Tvsekvyv tate netta-kvcckv em vruecicit omvyenken
   and caused broken days to go about among the men.
4. Tvsekvyv, cuku-lice elkv-vhuske emvhunkvtkv hvyomvteket
   and the men, and those interned in the house, so great a number
   left of death
5. "Upunvkvn okvtetisos" vn kuhmit
   "He meant talk" they thought of me
6. Tak fettv tate vn cukulahken heevyofv,
   My dooryard they two have come in when I see
7. "Muntos komit es vm ahlvpvtke estvmahet os," maket omes ce.
   So it is, I think, and am greatly satisfied, so he says:
8. Momen hvyomate?
   And now.
9. Pun cuku-pericvlke fullvranet omes.
   Our visitors will go about among us.
10. Momen ometo estomis.
    Even if that shall be.

[84a] See p. 609.
[84b] This system has the following peculiarities: v=á (a obscure); r=ł (surd l); e=ĭ; i=aĭ; c=tc.

11. Mvnnetvlke afvcketv eten haye omet.
    The young sporting among themselves.
12. Etepolice omis mome ocet omes.
    Laughing at each other they ofttimes do.
13. Mv tat momen umekares;
    That must not be.
14. "Vnen ukhoyis omes" komvranat ocet ometokv,
    "They probably mean me" because they may think.
15. Mvt momen umekares maket omesce.
    That must not be, so he says.
16. Munkv este e vhericet.
    Therefore the people must be careful of themselves.
17. Tak kaket umvres;
    As they two sit down;
18. Momen enhesse take em vlaket unt on omatehkvn.
    And if their friends shall come to them.
19. Humpetv hulwakusat en kvlepet.
    Victuals no matter how humble, you must break with them.
20. Umvranet omes komis maket omesce.
    Is the way I want it to be, so he says.
21. Momen hvyomate.
    And now.
22. Este en hesse take.
    Person's friends.
23. Hupvye estvmahen sehokvteto estomis.
    Although they two may have stood very far away.
24. Hvyomat em vcukuperet.
    If they are now visiting them.
25. Em fullet unt on omatehkvn.
    And going about among them.
26. Vhericet vseket.
    Take care to shake hands with them.
27. Em vpelet.
    Laugh with him.
28. Etem punahoyet omvres.
    Talk with him they should.
29. Maket omesce.
    So he says.
30. Momen hvyomate.
    And now.
31. Vmvculke sehokof.
    My old people when they two stood.
32. Heyvt em afvcketvt omvtetis.
    Although this was their amusement.
33. Vntatehkvn es cvhuse ome hakvtet unt omis.
    And although I have about forgotten it.

34. Hvyomat vhuckapkuse tayate.
   Now that which will at least resemble it.
35. Afvcketv hayit.
   Amusement I shall make.
36. Hvyomate tak kakin.
   And I too shall sit.
37. Vm estomvranet omes komis maket osce.
   Until it shall happen as it may, is my purpose, so he says.
38. Momen cuku-lice tate afvcketv tat.
   And the interned-in-the-house, amusement.
39. En hayvrabvyet omes, maketos.
   For them I shall provide, so he says.
40. Munkv cuku-lice a.
   Therefore the interned in the house.
41. Awet estomet em vculvke tate em afvcketvt omvte.
   They must come up, how their old ones that were, their amusement was.
42. En kerket ometokv.
   As it is known to them.
43. A awet vsehoket umvres maket omesce.
   They must come up and stand by it, so he says!

FREE TRANSLATION

I deemed it proper for our people, and a few days since caused
notice (broken days) to be given out among them; and when I see so
many men and women who have been spared from death and who
have heeded my notice, and come into the public square, I am greatly
pleased, he says.   And now we will have visitors coming to be with
us to enjoy with us these exercises.   We are glad to have them and
when they come, let there be no loud and boisterous laughing indulged in by our young people, lest the visitors construe such hilarity
as having been excited by their appearance and thereby be made to
feel embarrassed.   This must not be.   Our people therefore are enjoined to keep close watch over themselves, doing nothing that the
visitor might become offended at while we are here.   And if friends
shall come to your camp, you are enjoined to set before them such
scanty table fare as you are able to offer, be it ever so little.

You will doubtless be visited by friends living in distant parts
of the country; when they shall come you are asked to give them the
glad hand of friendship, laugh and talk with, and make them feel
perfectly welcome; this is my desire.   And now, when my old people
practiced their old customs in their entirety, the purpose for which
we meet here to-day was their joy and glory.   And although I have
well-nigh forgotten those beloved customs, I shall at least attempt
a semblance of them as best I may, and continue in the performance

to the end, so he says.   I propose to provide some amusement for our
women, so he says.   So I enjoin upon our women that they promptly
take their places; and as they understand the custom of our fore-
bears, they are asked to carry them out on this occasion, so he says.

During the busk names and titles different from those ordinarily
used were employed.   The women were called Hōmpita haya ("food
preparers"), or Tcukole'idji ("having a house").   This last term is
said to have been extended also to the children—that is, it included
all of those who remained in the houses instead of going to war
or the chase.   According to Cook it was applied in Tukabahchee
only to the four women who acted as leaders in the women's dance.
It was very bad form to refer to a woman or to women by the common terms.   In important speeches the people of the Raccoon clan
often said "I am of the Shawanogis," and this term also extended
to related clans like the Potato and Fox.   This applied particularly
to Tukabahchee and was based on the close friendship between the
Tukabahchee and the Shawnee.   According to Alindja, one of the
best Tukabahchee authorities, it was extended really to the whole
of Tukabahchee town, the term Tciloki bringing about a separation.
The Raccoon clan at Tukabahchee also called themselves Isti mikági
doiyàt ("chiefs that we are") or isti tcilokogi doiyàt ("Tcilokis
that we are").   The towns often had particular busk names.   The
Abihka would be known as Abihka nági, the Coweta as Kawita
mahma'ya, the Kasihta as Kasihta łako.   The Okchai called themselves by that name and the almost as common term Łałogàlga.
The Okfuskee and Tulsa people called themselves Kos i'stàgi ("people
of Coosa").   The Pákàn tallahassee used the word Pákana.

SHAMANISM AND MEDICINE

GENERAL REMARKS

Just as among the beings and objects in nature there were certain
which possessed or acquired exceptional supernatural powers, so
there were certain men who were possessed of such power or were
mediums for its expression.   They were also versed in the powers
possessed by other created things and hence were partly prophets
or soothsayers and partly doctors, while some of them occupied
official or semiofficial positions and became priests.

Both men and women could be doctors.   Swan, in fact, states
that women were employed more frequently than men.[85]   If this
means that the female doctors were more numerous than the male
he is probably incorrect, since very little is said of female doctors
by anyone else, and I have heard little about them personally.
Perhaps Swan had reference in part to the common practitioners,

---

[85] Schoolcraft, Ind. Tribes, vol. v, p. 270.

persons who did not assume to have much supernatural power but were none the less acquainted with remedies and were called in in cases of minor importance. It is likely that such persons existed in almost every large family group and probably they were more often women than men. The old women were naturally the midwives. As with us there were home remedies known to almost every one, still others known only to certain of the old people, and finally medicines and medical processes which were the sole property of the various grades of shamans.

THE "KNOWERS"

The principal individuals who combined medical and priestly functions were the kīlas or "knowers," usually called by the whites "prophets," and the priests or doctors proper, known as alektca, or medicine makers, hilis-haya. There were only a few of the former and they are said always to have been men, but the second were more numerous, and had more to do directly with healing. While the kīla might also be a good doctor his work in that line was generally confined to a determination of the kind of disease with which the sick person was afflicted.[86] He might best be described as the diagnostician, though his diagnosis consisted merely in the examination of an article of clothing belonging to the sick man. From this he claimed to be able to determine the nature of the disorder and he sent back word accordingly. Of course, many doctors, partly from having seen so many cases diagnosed by the kīla, would be so expert that they would not ordinarily need to refer to him. The kīla was something of a clairvoyant and probably a juggler also, and about this class many wonderful tales are told. It was thought that the younger of twins was likely to make an efficient kīla. Natchez and Cherokee informants stated that twins would be prophets until they were 8 or 10 years old, when the gift would leave them, but if they were carefully watched they would become prophets when they grew up. My Cherokee interpreter had a brother and sister who were twins. His father, a man often outlawed, said that they frequently warned him of impending trouble. It was thought that triplets might know still more. In one case triplets told their father, who had been acquitted several times before the courts, that the next time he would be hung, and in consequence he took good care to keep out of trouble. It was the kīla who learned events from birds as narrated on page 496. He could foretell death, sickness, or crime, and in the last case he would sometimes send his dogs to punish the offenders.

---

[86] The people of Tukabahchee and neighboring towns believed that Megillis Hadjo [miko hilis hadjo?], the prophet of Tukabahchee, met by Hitchcock in 1842, had control over the elements and could make the weather pleasant or disagreeable. They thought he could see into the future and predict events, and in cases of sickness he was frequently called upon to divine and to define the cause.—Hitchcock, Ms. notes.

It is asserted that a prophet could tell a person where to find a stolen horse; could shorten a road, making it draw together as if it were made of rubber; could make beads, finger rings, or bullets swim on the surface of the water; could throw a bead into the middle of a stream, make it swim toward shore, and cause another bead to swim out to meet it. He could determine whether a person's life was to be long or short by setting up a stake and making another object move toward it "by his power." If this reached the stake, the person's life would be long; if it fell short of it his life would be short.

Near Yahola station, on the Midland Valley Railroad, lived an old kĭla from whom the station derived its name. He had cleared out spaces around his house said to represent the square grounds of the different Creek towns (pl. 13, c).

The Texas Alabama tell of a prophet who stopped rain by fasting and putting medicine on the water of a creek. Another stopped a storm which was brought on when his companion shot a buzzard, mistaking it for a turkey. On another occasion some people were in the middle of a lake and were surrounded on all sides by enemies who had lighted fires all about on the banks so that they could not escape during the night. However, a prophet among the people on the water made it rain, thereby putting out the fires, and enabling them to get through the lines of their enemy. Still another prophet brought on rain in the following manner. He sent a boy out to catch fish, and when they were brought he dived with them to the bottom of a creek and gave them to certain long, horned snakes living there which go under both the water and the land. These snakes are called in Alabama tcinto săktco and have been described on page 494. Then these snakes made the rain fall. More often, however, rain making is ascribed to a separate set of rain makers.

Although he confounds knowers and shamans, it must be the former to whom Bossu refers in the following words:

"The savages have much confidence in their medicine men; the cabin of the jugglers (jongleur) is covered with skins which serve him as a covering or clothing. He enters it entirely naked and begins to pronounce some words which none understands: it is, says he, to invoke the spirit; after which he rises, cries, is agitated, appears beside himself, and water pours from all parts of his body.

"The cabin shakes, and those present think that it is the presence of the Spirit; the language which he speaks in these invocations has nothing in common with the language of the savages; it is only through a heated imagination that these charlatans have found the means of making it pass for a divine language, it is thus in all times that the most clever have duped the others."[87]

---

[87] Bossu, Nouv. Voy., vol. II, p. 58, note.

The "Fasters" or Doctors

The doctors or priests—at least a great majority of them—belonged to a class of learned men called isti poskálgi ("fasting men"), already referred to, who had received their training in certain schools of higher learning, if we may so denominate them. This training was called by the same name, pōskita, "to fast," as that given to the great town ceremonial, because in both fasting was an essential element. It was generally undertaken in summer when a person can lie out of doors comfortably and proceeds about as follows, according to Jackson Lewis, who had taken five courses, in this aboriginal college. From one to four young men—Lewis did not remember parties of more than four—would go into the town and engage some old Indian who was known to have passed through the course and was prepared to teach them. Then all repaired together to a stream of water, usually a densely wooded creek bottom where they were not likely to be observed. As a further protection they threw together boughs so as to screen themselves still more completely, for during their stay there they did not want to be so much as seen. The "red root," miko hoyanïdja, was dug by each candidate, pounded up and put into a pot already provided, and the pot filled with water. Then the instructor came in and blew into the medicine through a cane. After blowing into it and singing over it he went away. This was supposed to give the medicine virtue. Then the novice drank great quantities of medicine at intervals of an hour or more, so arranging it that by noon he would have taken it four separate times. At noon the instructor came back and then began to tell the novice either by words or songs some of the most elementary things he had to learn. After talking for some time he went away. When the sun was just above the western horizon he came back and gave more instruction and left the man in the woods again.

The first thing that would be taught was how to treat gunshot wounds. There were three ways of treating these: (1) For flesh wounds, (2) for bowel wounds, (3) for head wounds. The instructor would tell what to do and what songs to sing in order to give virtue to the medicine they made for the wounds. Then the instructor said, "You sing this. Sing it as I have sung it to you." Sometimes these are merely recited formulas. When the novice had repeated as best he could what the instructor had told him the instructor criticized, and corrected him where he had made mistakes. Then he instructed him again and said, "Now go over it as I have." He did not stop because his pupil had repeated it correctly once but made him go over it often later, because unless it was gone over in just such a manner it would not be effective when used. After this he would teach the novice the proper treatment for any disease that the latter might desire to learn about. This instruction was continued for four successive days. Then the novice stopped because the teacher thought it better for him to think these things over and repeat them to himself for a while before learning more. After a month or two, during which the novice went back to the town, he could return to the woods and take another course. There were only slight variations between the methods of instruction of different teachers. Few ever took a complete course. After the fifth or sixth 4-day period one could ask the teacher to put him through the 8-day session, and after that he could ask the teacher to put him through the 12-day session, which was the last. There were very few teachers because very few had passed through the 12-day course. This instruction seems to have required fasting and isolation from noise because nothing was written and everything must be imprinted on the mind. Noises would disturb the process. After the first 4-day session had been gone through a blanket was thrown about the novice and water was poured upon hot stones inside of this until steam was raised, and after the novice was thoroughly steamed he went to bathe in a cold creek. Then he went home feeling very hungry but unable to eat much because his stomach was drawn up from fasting and the frequent taking of the red root emetic. None of the other tribes with which Lewis was acquainted had anything similar to this. After the education had been completed the old teacher would dig a trench in the ground, put a cane in the novice's mouth so that he might breathe through it, cover him with earth, put leaves over all, and set fire to them. Then he would order the novice to get up and, having done so, he was ready for any emergency in life. Lewis knew of many who had not gone as far as he but pretended to be proficient in all branches. One who had gone as far as himself was entitled to embellish his headdress with a feather of the horned owl, "which many fellows who actually know little wear to-day." It also entitled him to wear a buzzard feather, the insignia of the man able to treat gunshot wounds. Lewis once cured his son, who had been shot through the breast so that the air seemed to be coming out of the vent. The buzzard's feather was used because that feather was employed in cleaning out the wound before treating it. Lewis could appropriately wear a fox's skin, because he could cure a snake bite. These insignia ought to be worn only when a body of people is going to war or is collected on account of some danger. They served to single out the persons who were to be approached in case of trouble. If you find an Indian with a streak of red paint in one corner of the mouth extending down to the side it means he is capable of treating a person injured in an affray. The fox's skin is worn because foxes catch and eat snakes, showing that they, like the wearer of the fox skin, can conquer them. A person who can cure a snake bite also has a tobacco pouch made of opossum skin, because an opossum can kill and eat a snake like a fox. In early times these men were always preparing young people for war, and, as much of this work had to be done at night, fine eyesight was requisite. The old teacher also taught his pupil how to trail and locate an enemy and he believed he was teaching him how to acquire extraordinary vision at night. That was why the latter used an owl feather.

When the novice fasted it was expected that he would have a dream (or vision). Lewis himself dreamed that a very clear, beautiful day had dawned upon him and a number of white birds were coming toward him. When his teacher heard it he said, "That is a very good sign, a clear day and white birds. You will be a good doctor of gunshot wounds."

The only other account of this poskita known to me is the following, from Hawkins:

"At the age of from fifteen to seventeen, this ceremony is usually performed. It is called Boos-ke-tau, in like manner as the annual Boosketau of the nation. A youth of the proper age gathers two handsfull of the Sou-watch-cau, a very bitter root, which he eats a whole day; then he steeps the leaves in water and drinks it. In the dusk of the evening, he eats two or three spoonfuls of boiled grits. This is repeated for four days, and during this time he remains in a house. The Sou-watch-cau has the effect of intoxicating and maddening. The fourth day he goes out, but must put on a pair of new moccasins (Stil-la-pica). For twelve moons, he abstains from eating bucks, except old ones, and from turkey cocks, fowls, peas and salt. During this period he must not pick his ears, or scratch his head with his fingers, but use a small stick. For four moons he must have a fire to himself, to cook his food, and a little girl, a virgin, may cook for him; his food is boiled grits. The fifth moon, any person may cook for him, but he must serve himself first, and use one spoon and pan. Every new moon, he drinks for four days the possau, (button snake-root,) an emetic, and abstains for these days, from all food, except in the evening, a little boiled grits, (humpetuh hutke.) The twelfth moon, he performs for four days, what he commenced with on the first. The fifth day, he comes out of his house, gathers corn cobs, burns them to ashes, and with these, rubs his body all over. At the end of this moon, he sweats under blankets, then goes into water, and this ends the ceremony. This ceremony is sometimes extended to four, six, or eight moons, or even to twelve days only, but the course is the same.

"During the whole of this ceremony, the physic is administered by the Is-te-puc-cau-chau thluc-co, (great leader,) who in speaking of a youth under initiation, says, 'I am physicing him,' (Boo-se-ji-jite saut li-to-misce-cha,) or 'I am teaching him all that is proper for him to know,' (nauk o-mul-gau e-muc-e-thli-jite saut litomise cha.) The youth, during this initiation, does not touch any one except young persons, who are under a like course with himself, and if he dreams, he drinks the possau." [88]

Those who had gone through with this training were held in high esteem, and there appears to have been no fast for persons not intending to become doctors except at the great annual ceremony. In lore of this kind the Shawnee are believed to be very rich. The following quotation from Adair shows that, in spite of Lewis's claim that this ordeal was peculiar to the Creeks, a similar institution existed among the Chickasaw, except that admission was secured through inheritance:

"*Ishtohoollo* is the name of all their priestly order, and their pontifical office descends by inheritance to the eldest: those friend-towns, which are firmly confederated in their exercises and plays, never have more than one *Archi-magus* at a time . . . They, who have the least knowledge of Indian affairs, know, that the martial virtues of the savages, obtains them titles of distinction; but yet their old men, who could scarcely correct their transgressing wives, much less go to war, and perform those difficult exercises, that are essentially needful in an active warrior, are often promoted to the pontifical dignity, and have great power over the people, by the pretended sanctity of the office" . . .[89]

It appears that this order of "magi" were the custodians not only of medical secrets but of secrets supposed to be of value in warfare, of the sacred myths, and of various branches of learning.

At the head of the priesthood in each town was the hilis-haya or "medicine maker," who communicated the necessary spiritual qualities to the medicines at the annual busk, had general charge of the public health, protected all from ghosts, and so on. While fitness was regarded rather than descent in selecting this high priest, some towns at least preferred to take him from a certain clan, oftenest the clan of the miko. According to the last miko of Chiaha the medicine maker of that town was elected for four years only, at the end of which period he might be reelected or displaced. Speaking of the Chickasaw in the middle of the eighteenth century, Adair says: "the title of *old beloved men*, or *archimagi*, is still hereditary in the *panther*, or *tyger family*." [90] Bartram calls this functionary the "high priest." The Creeks "have," he says, "an ancient high-priest, with juniors in

[88] Ga. Hist. Soc. Colls., vol. III, pp. 78-79.   [90] Ibid., p. 31.
[89] Adair, Hist. Am. Inds., p. 81.

every town and tribe. The high-priest is a person of great power and consequence in the state. He always sits in council, and his advice in affairs of war is of the greatest weight and importance, and he or one of his disciples always attends a war party." "It sometimes happens," he adds, "that the king is war-chief and high-priest, and then his power is very formidable and sometimes dangerous to the liberty of citizens, and he must be a very cunning man if the tomahawk or rifle do not cut him short." [91]

The following statement by the same writer bears out what Jackson Lewis says regarding the insignia of graduates and adds some details.

"The junior priests or students constantly wear the mantle or robe, which is white; and they have a great owl skin cased and stuffed very ingeniously, so well executed, as almost to represent the living bird, having large sparkling glass beads, or buttons, fixed in the head for eyes; this ensign of wisdom and divination, they wear sometimes as a crest on the top of the head, at other times the image fits on the arm, or is borne on the hand. These bachelors are also distinguishable from the other people by their taciturnity, grave and solemn countenance, dignified step, and singing to themselves songs or hymns, in a low sweet voice, as they stroll about the town." [92]

They were, of course, men who had taken some courses in medicine. Regarding the headdress it is instructive to compare those in some of Le Moyne's drawings of the Florida Indians.[92a]

A graduate in medicine, or at least one of a certain degree, could paint a black circle round each eye when he went out at night. This was in imitation of the markings of the raccoon and signified that he could see anything in the dark. If a man had been killed at night a doctor having this power would paint these circles about his eyes and track the murderer right to his own house. He could see his tracks "like a spider's web" and follow them. One of the means for attaining this ability to see in the dark was by using the "star medicine" (kodjodjámbà hiliswa). According to Silas Jefferson, a man with a "skunk's pouch" was considered a great medicine man capable of charming any kind of animal. There was no uniformity, however, in the costumes worn by doctors. Outside of certain generally understood insignia each dressed to suit himself. One doctor is said to have carried big spiders and snakes about in order to scare people.

Frequent scratchings were resorted to by the medicine men that they might keep in health. A graduate in medicine was not allowed to eat catfish, for if he did it was thought that the fish bones would cause weevil to bore into the beans.

---

[91] Trans. Am. Eth. Soc., vol. III, p. 24.   [92a] Le Moyne, Jacques, Narrative, Trans., Boston, 1875.
[92] Bartram, Travels, p. 502.

METHODS OF PRACTICING

The method of bestowing medical treatment seems to have changed progressively after first contact with the whites, the religious features becoming less and less pronounced and the features connected with the administration of the medicine more and more important. Adair's account of the performance among the Chickasaw in the middle of the eighteenth century is as follows:

"When the Indian physicians visit their supposed irreligious patients, they approach them in a bending posture, with their rattling calabash, preferring that sort to the North-American gourds: and in that bent posture of body, they run two or three times round the sick person, contrary to the course of the sun, invoking God as already exprest. Then they invoke the raven; and mimic his croaking voice . . . They also place a bason of cold water with some pebbles in it on the ground, near the patient, then they invoke the fish, because of its cool element, to cool the heat of the fever. Again, they invoke the eagle, (Ooóle) they solicit him as he soars in the heavens, to bring down refreshing things for their sick, and not to delay them, as he can dart down upon the wing, quick as a flash of lightning. They are so tedious on this subject, that it would be a task to repeat it: however, it may be needful to observe, that they chuse the eagle because of its supposed communicative virtues; and that it is according to its Indian name, a cherubimical emblem, and the king of birds, of prodigious strength, swiftness of wing, majestic stature, and loving its young ones so tenderly, as to carry them on its back, and teach them to fly.[93]

Of the Chickasaw of a later date we read:

"When they are sick, they send for a doctor, (they have several among them,) after looking at the sick a-while, the family leave him and the sick alone. He then commences singing and shaking a gourd over the patient. This is done, not to cure, but to find out what is the matter or disease: as the doctor sings several songs, he watches closely the patient, and finds out which song pleased: then he determines what the disease is: he then uses herbs, roots, steaming, and conjuring: the doctor frequently recommends to have a large feast: (which they call Tonsh-pa-shoo-phah;) if the Indian is tolerably well off, and is sick for two or three weeks, they may have two or three Tonsh-pa-shoo-phahs.[94] They eat, dance, and sing at a great rate,

---

[93] Adair, Hist. Am. Inds., pp. 173-174.

[94] Tonsh-pa-shoo-phah is tanshi ặt pishofa, "the corn is hulled."

at these feasts; the doctors say that it raises the spirits of the sick, and weakens the evil spirit.[95]

Today they call these dances by a shortened form of the name, Pishofa dances; they will be discussed at length in a subsequent paper.

The later Creek performance was much tamer than the ancient ritual. If a person were sick and his family knew what medicine to send for they did so; if not they got the physician's advice and procured the herbs, and other things he ordered. The pot was laid out for him with the medicine plants near it and beside all a cane for him to blow through, also a chair for him to sit in and a small gift to encourage him. Four root stalks or branches of the medicine were generally used, and in gathering these the doctor sometimes faced east and sometimes one of the other cardinal points in accordance with the nature of the remedy. Bark and branches were generally taken from the east sides of the trees. The medicine was piled into the pot at the direction of the physician, along with water, after which he blew into it through the cane four separate times after as many repetitions of a sacred fromula suited to the kind of disease which he supposed the patient had contracted. He came four successive mornings, allowing the gift to remain where it had been placed until the fourth, when he took it with him. This gift might be some cloth—perhaps 10 yards of calico—money, a handkerchief, or, if the doctor were a woman, a shawl. Money has been given only in late times.

The points of the compass are frequently named in these formulæ. The circuit is always sinistral or contraclockwise, and according to the best information I could get it usually begins with the north and ends with the east because the east is associated with life or the renewal of it. According to one informant, however, it ended with the south, and there may have been variations in the formulæ because the colors attached to these points are admitted to vary. One of my best informants stated that they were either: North (honeta), green; west (akàlatkà), red; south (wahàla), black; and east (hàsosa), white; or else north, red; west, green; south, black; and east, white. The black is said to stand for the shade or something of that sort, but it does not seem natural that it should be to the south. The table following contains seven lists of colors applied to the cardinal points by several different bodies of Creeks, and a list from the Cherokee band of Natchez, obtained from several different authorities.

---

[95] Schoolcraft, Ind. Tribes, vol. i, p. 310.

	North	West	South	East
Chekilli, speech to Oglethorpe (Kasihta).	Red and yellow.	Black	Blue	White.[1]
Tuggle, Ms	Red	Yellow	Black	Do.[2]
Lasley Cloud, through F. Speck (Tuskegee).	Black	...do	Red	Do.[3]
Big Jack (Hilibi)	Green	Red	Black	Do.
	Red	Green	...do	Do.
Z. Cook (Tukabahchee)	Black	...do	White	Red.
Silas Jefferson (Tuskegee)	Green	Black	Brown	Yellow.
Texas Alabama	Yellow	...do	Red	White.
Watt Sam (Natchez)	...do	...do	...do	Do.

[1] Gatschet, Creek Mig. Leg., vol. I, p. 245.
[2] Ms., Bur. Amer. Ethn.
[3] Mem. Am. Anth. Assn., vol. II, p. 23.

Here red and yellow is each applied to the north in three lists, and black and green in two; black is applied to the west in four lists, yellow and green in two each, and red in one; black is applied to the south in three cases, brown in one, red in three, and blue and white in one each; white is applied to the east in seven cases and yellow and red in one each. In conjuring for the dog disease the cardinal points were faced in the same order as that first given, ending with the east, but no colors were mentioned. In others neither the points nor the colors occurred. When he blew into the medicine, however, the doctor almost always faced east. An Alabama doctor would sing one verse of the medicine formula and call upon the north, sing another and call upon the west, sing a third and call upon the south, and sing a fourth and call upon the east. Then he would blow into the medicine and do the same thing again, passing around the circuit four times and blowing into the medicine after each circuit. Afterwards the patient was given some medicine to drink, and, wetting the ends of his fingers in it, the doctor rubbed some on the patient's ears, arms, legs, breast, and in fact his whole body. The north was referred to as the "yellow water," the west as "the black water," the south as "the red water," and the east as "the white water," and they were enumerated in that order, as in the table above.

According to my Natchez informant, himself a medicine man, the sick person must be laid with his head to the east. It was like administering poison, he affirmed, to turn the heads of the sick in any other direction, because "the east meant long life and good fortune while the west meant short life." Bark, roots, and other portions of trees or bushes which entered into the remedies were taken from the east side. If a person became weak and emaciated, his name might be changed.

Blood letting and sucking were frequently resorted to. Swan says that the Indians sometimes believed that they had been super- naturally shot by enemies hundreds of miles away and would then consult a doctress. "The cunning woman tells them that what they have apprehended is verily true, and proceeds to examine and make the cure. In these cases, scratching or cupping is the remedy; or, as is often the case, sucking the affected part with her mouth, she produces to their view some fragment of a bullet, or piece of a wad, which she had purposely concealed in her mouth to confirm the truth of what she had asserted; after this, a few magic draughts of their physic must be administered, and the patient is made whole."[96] Jackson Lewis said that pricks were sometimes made over the affected part with a little piece of glass. The large end of a short piece of cow horn was then placed over them and a quantity of blood sucked out through a hole pierced in the small end. Silas Jefferson states that he was once treated by a snake doctor who simply chewed up a bit of root and, holding it in his mouth, sucked out the poison. Next day he was perfectly restored. But unlike the former European practice, blood letting was not resorted to in cases of fever.[97]

Eakins says that bandages and lints were applied in many cases. He continues: "The success with which they treat gunshot wounds, cuts, &c., is generally attributed to the care of the physician. The Creeks never amputate. They are skilful in the use of splints. For removing the wounded they use the litter."[97]

Adair furnishes some information regarding the treatment of those wounded in war.

"The Indians . . . build a small hut at a considerable distance from the houses of the village, for every one of their warriors wounded in war, and confine them there . . . for the space of four moons, including that moon in which they were wounded, as in the case of their women after travail: and they keep them strictly separate, lest the impurity of the one should prevent the cure of the other. The reputed prophet, or divine physician, daily pays them a due attendance, always invoking Yo He Wah to bless the means they apply on the sad occasion; which is chiefly mountain allum, and medicinal herbs, always injoyning a very abstemious life, prohibiting them women and salt in particular, during the time of the cure, or sanctifying the reputed sinners. Like the Israelites, they firmly believe that safety, or wounds, etc., immediately proceed from the pleased, or angry deity, for their virtuous, or vicious conduct, in observing, or violating the divine law.

"In this long space of purification, each patient is allowed only a superannuated woman to attend him, who is past the temptations of

[96] Schoolcraft, Ind. Tribes, vol. v, p. 271.   [97] Ibid., vol. I, p. 274.

sinning with men, lest the introduction of a young one should either seduce him to folly; or she having committed it with others—or by not observing her appointed time of living apart from the rest, might thereby defile the place, and totally prevent the cure. But what is yet more surprising in their physical, or rather theological regimen, is, that the physician is so religiously cautious of not admitting polluted persons to visit any of his patients, lest the defilement should retard the cure, or spoil the warriors, that before he introduces any man, even any of their priests, who are married according to the law, he obliges him to assert either by a double affirmative, or by two negatives, that he has not known even his own wife, in the space of the last natural day.'' [99]

In earlier times it is said that the doctors claimed to have intercourse with good or bad spirits, but this personal side of the influences which they controlled appears to have gradually fallen out so that they were later of a general magic nature rather than through personal assisting spirits.

The "white day" and the "white smoke" were expressions used in medical formulæ or incantations. It is said that the term "white day" was specifically applied to the treatment given to a man wounded in war because by "giving him the white day" the doctor was prolonging his life. Two Creeks told General Hitchcock that doctors sometimes prescribed gifts to the tcokofa as a means of cure. This suggests a sanctity connected with that building similar to the sanctity attaching to the Natchez temple.

"If the physician fails in his cure," says Swan, "he will ascribe it to the cats or dogs that may be about the house; and they are either killed instantly, or sent out of the neighborhood. If after all the patient dies, the chance is two to one that the doctor is considered as a witch or sorcerer, influenced by the devil, and is pursued, beaten, and sometimes killed by the surviving relations; but if successful in restoring the patient to health, he is paid almost his own price for his services, in skins or cattle.''[1] This dangerous side of shamanism is noted by Bossu and other writers and mentioned by some of my informants.[2]

Another method of doctoring was by sweat baths. These were generally taken in a small lodge composed of blankets thrown over a framework of slender poles. When prepared to take a sweat bath they heated stones, carried them into the lodge and threw on them water which had first been doctored by being blown into through a cane. Some Indians were taking sweat baths regularly as late as 1914.

Doctors sometimes engaged in supernatural fights with one another. Upon one occasion a doctor showed his power by throwing his hand-

[99] Adair, Hist. Am. Inds., p. 125.   [1] Schoolcraft, Ind. Tribes, vol. v, p. 271.
[2] Bossu, Nouv. Voy., vol. II, p. 59.

kerchief at a tree up which it ran like a squirrel. His opponent then produced a number of centipedes which ran about everywhere but hurt no one. The first then began to try to reach his antagonist in the shapes of various animals, sometimes burrowing under the earth to get at him. Finally, however, the other created a centipede which bit him in the hand and killed him.

As noted above, Shawnee doctors were in particular esteem among the Creeks, an esteem shared by all the other peoples in contact with them. Even the Texas Alabama know the reputed powers of Shawnee doctors well and told me the following story regarding the accomplishments of one of them.

Some Alabama were once traveling along with this doctor. One night they heard what sounded like the whinnying of horses. The Shawnee told them, however, that it was produced by some Comanche Indians, and when day came they discovered four of these Indians in a tree. By his medicine he caused these persons to fall asleep and then tumble to the ground without waking up. In a river bend near by was a great crowd of Comanche, but the Shawnee rendered himself and his companions invisible, so that the Comanche did not see them, and they passed safely on.

It was claimed that when a doctor died all of the medicine he had taken ran away from him in the forms of animals of various kinds, such as lizards and snakes. He died because or when these creatures became too powerful for him. As long as he kept his power over them they remained in him and were his strength. This is from Creek sources and is confirmed in substance by what is said about witchcraft, to which we will turn presently.

The following from Adair leads one to suppose that the medicine maker and other doctors whose positions were official or semiofficial were forced to undergo a special fast and purification before taking their posts, but I have no other evidence regarding it.

"The Indian priests and prophets are initiated by unction. The Chikkasah some time ago set apart some of their old men of the religious order. They first obliged them to sweat themselves for the space of three days and nights, in a small green hut, made on purpose, at a considerable distance from any dwelling; through a scrupulous fear to contracting pollution by contact, or from the effluvia of polluted people—and a strong desire of secreting their religious mysteries. During that interval, they are allowed to eat nothing but green tobacco, nor to drink any thing except warm water, highly imbittered with the button-snake-root, to cleanse their bodies, and prepare them to serve in their holy, or beloved office, before the divine essence, whom during this preparation they constantly invoke by his essential name, as before described. After which, their priestly garments and ornaments, mentioned under a former argument, page 84, are put on, and then bear's oil is poured upon their head."[3]

Certain things were done to ward off misfortune before any actual ill effects had been experienced—an aboriginal application of the ounce of prevention axiom. Hitci pȧkpȧgi, the "old man's tobacco," was kept on hand as a protection against the souls of the dead, and a great deal was paid for it. Some of the busk medicines were carried home to help guard the family from harm during the succeeding year, and just outside of and above the door of one of my informants was hung the adilōga or mixed medicine used at that time, while the other medicine, the miko hoyanīdja, was hung just to one side within. This is said to be a common custom with the old-time Indians. At intervals it was thought best to scratch the grown-up men in order to let out bad blood, supposed to have become clogged up inside of them. An Okfuskee Indian told me that he had only recently performed such an operation on 13 men at Nuyaka. These were adults; usually only the young people were scratched.

When a hunting party set out and as soon as it had gotten to the edge of the town, an old man would fall back behind the rest, chew up some sassafras or angelica root, and spit it out toward each of the cardinal points four times. Then he would walk back, singing, and do the same thing four times more. This ceremony was supposed to counteract anything that the spirits of the living might do to injure the hunt by thinking or talking too mich about the hunters or by making sport of them. When they came into the settlement on their return they built a fire in a place apart by themselves and sang and danced the stomp dance there all night to prevent the fires they had lighted during the hunt from creating diseases among the families.[4]

The following performance belongs in the same category as the phenomena just considered.

"In the Summer-season of the year 1746 [says Adair], I chanced to see the Indians playing at a house of the former Mississippi-Nachee, on one of their old sacred musical instruments. It pretty much resembled the Negroe-Banger in shape but far exceeded it in dimensions: for it was about five feet long, and a foot wide on the head-part of the board, with eight strings made out of the sinews of a large buffalo. But they were so unskillful in acting the part of the Lyrick, that the *Loache*, or prophet who held the instrument between his feet, and along side of his chin, took one end of the bow, whilst a lusty fellow held the other; by sweating labour they scraped out such harsh jarring sounds, as might have been reasonably ex-

[3] Adair, Hist. Am. Inds.. p. 122.
[4] Further information on hunting ceremonies will be found on pp. 444–445.

pected by a soft ear, to have been sufficient to drive out the devil
if he lay anywhere hid in the house. When I afterward asked him the
name, and the reason of such a strange method of diversion, he told
me the dance was called *Keetla Ishto Hoollo,* 'a dance to, or before,
the great holy one;'[5] that it kept off evil spirits, witches, and wizards,
from the red people; and enabled them to ordain elderly men to officiate in holy things, as the exigency of the times required.

"He who danced to it, kept his place and posture, in a very exact
manner, without the least perceivable variation: yet by the prodigious working of his muscles and nerves, he in about half an hour,
foamed in a very extraordinary manner, and discontinued it propor-
tionally, till he recovered himself."[6]

The Indians were and still are satisfied that their system of doctoring
is vastly superior to that used by the whites, but the system of white
doctoring with which the Indians were formerly familiar can not be
said to represent upon the whole a very perfect development of
the medical art, and there has been more than one occasion for them
to complain like the Chickasaw of Adair's time of the performances of
"civilized" surgeons. The success of native remedies was due in
part without doubt to the real medicinal virtues of the plants used,
in part to the good effects of such a simple assistant as sweat bathing,
and perhaps to a greater extent to the power of suggestion. Swan
was, however, quite right in saying that the results were not as
certain as had commonly been reported.[7]

WEATHER CONTROLLERS

Besides the healers there were men and women who professed to
be able to cause rain or drought, to blow away the clouds, or "blow
the rain" as they described it. When a storm was coming up an
Alabama doctor would blow into his clasped hands, rub them together,
and then wave them upward and outward. Then, even if it rained,
the wind would not blow. The same person claimed to be able to
cause rain or drought.

Hitchcock says: "There are people who affect to think they can
make it rain and they go to a piece of shallow water and roll and wal-
low in the muddy water every morning for four mornings in succession. They have a pot of medicine in one hand and a buffalo
tail in the other and sing continually for an hour or more. During
this time they take black drink every morning."[8]

He also gives some interesting particulars regarding the meteoro
logical activities of Megillis Hadjo, the prophet or kĭla of Tukabah-

---

[5] Hĭia ishto holo, "dance of the spirit or spirits"; hĭia, "dance"; ishto, "big"; holo, what is "holy,
sacred," or "supernatural."

[6] Adair, Hist. Am. Inds., p. 175.

[7] Schoolcraft, Ind. Tribes, vol. v, p. 271.

[8] Hitchcock, Ms. notes.

chee town. "In the summer of 1840," he says, "there was a great drought in the country, threatening the destruction of the crops, and the old man was called upon to make it rain. After performing his ceremony for a time he published that he was about to be so successful that the country might be flooded, and he thought it best to desist, which he did. Last winter (1840–41) was very cold and the old man was requested to moderate the weather; the present winter (1841–42) is remarkably mild and the old man explains it by saying that he blew off the cold of last winter so far that it has not come back." [9]

Some interesting particulars regarding rain makers are also given us by Adair. According to him, these persons obtained rain by interceding through their conjurations with "the bountiful holy Spirit of Fire," by which he supposes they referred to the supreme deity of the southern Indians, although in fact it may have been the particular being presiding over thunder.[10] This power of intercession had been established in ancient times and was not exercised merely at the option of its possessor, but was a duty which he owed to the community and which the community could demand from him. If he failed he was likely to be shot dead because it was supposed that he really had the power but refused to exercise it, and was thus an enemy to the state. However, he frequently saved himself by laying the blame upon lay infractions of the sacred regulations or taboos— among them the payments which they owed to him—which rendered his best endeavors unavailing. If the drought were prolonged as much as two years, a council was held at which they did not fail to discover that the trouble was due to persistent violations of the taboos by certain individuals, who were then promptly dispatched. Too much rain might work as much to the harm of the rain maker as too little, Adair instancing a case of a Creek rain maker who was shot because the river overflowed the fields to a great height in the middle of August.[11] These men had a transparent stone "of supposed great power in assisting to bring down the rain, when it is put in a basin of water," and this power was supposed to have been passed down to this one from a stone to which the power had originally been committed. As usual, this stone could not be exposed to the gaze of the vulgar without losing mightily in efficacy.[12] The control of the rain maker extended only to the summer rains and not to those which fell in winter, and it was believed that this was also of supernatural ordination. The summer rain had to be sought for; the winter rain was given unsought. If the seasons were good, the rain maker was paid a certain proportion of each kind of food. It is amusing to note that, like the apologist for obsolescent institutions at the present day, the Chickasaw rain maker with whom Adair conversed took the ground "that though the former beloved speech

[9] Hitchcock, Ms. notes.
[10] Adair, Hist. Am. Inds., p. 85.
[11] Ibid., pp. 85–86.
[12] Ibid., pp. 86–87.

had a long time subsided, it was very reasonable they should still continue this their old beloved custom; especially as it was both profitable in supporting many of their helpless old beloved men, and very productive of virtue, by awing their young people from violating the ancient laws." [13]

There were others who claimed they could make the waters in swollen streams subside, and still another class of dew makers, who could also prevent the dew from falling. If there had been a dry spring someone might say, at the time of the first stomp dance, "There is a dew maker over yonder. Let us invite him to make dew for us." It is said that such a man could not assist anyone, even though he desired to do so, unless he were formally invited. The council having agreed, he would come over and go through with his incantations, and a treat was given him by way of payment. If, after this had been done, it still continued dry at the time of the next stomp dance, it might be suggested that a rain maker be called in. Eakins remarks dryly that "the weather, about the time of the distribution of the annuity, in some parts of the nation, falls under the scrutiny of the physic-makers." [13a] He probably means men of the above class.

According to early writers some doctors claimed to be able to control the thunder and lightning, but we are not informed whether they were a separate class or identical with one of those already mentioned. Bartram was present when a Seminole chief threatened one of the white traders that, if he did not comply with his requests, he would cause the thunder and lightning to descend upon his head and reduce his stores to ashes.

WITCHCRAFT

The great powers which doctors and graduates of the native schools generally enjoyed, while in theory capable of being exerted for the good of the community and the individuals composing it, might equally well be perverted to their injury or destruction. Jackson Lewis said that the same learned men who acted as instructors in medicine and the lore of the tribe generally could teach witchcraft, but he added that they advised against it, saying that it was only for mischief and that anyone who practiced it would eventually come to a dog's death, because witches were killed. But since such knowledge was known to reside in the great doctors and graduates and it was never certain that it would not be employed, these people were constantly open to suspicion, and, as Swan tells us in the quotation given above, a doctor whose patient died was apt to suffer from the imputation of witchcraft and be put to death himself. An Alabama informant told me that when he was a young man an old woman was accused of being a witch and cut to pieces. This sus-

---

[13] Adair, Hist. Am. Inds., pp. 84–94. [13a] Schoolcraft, Ind. Tribes, vol. I, p. 277

picion was also encouraged by the doctors themselves, who frequently attributed sickness to the doings of witches, and the public mind was kept wrought up to a condition of feverish excitement and fear by the most grewsome tales vouched for as absolute truth.

Says Stiggins:

"They are tinctured with superstition and believe anything of a marvelous report. As soon as it is announced that a man is acquainted with the work and dismal effects of the diabolical art, such as flying about the country far and near to poison such people as are inimical to him, or blowing and infusing a contagious air into a house in passing by it at night or into the nostrils and lungs of a particular person while asleep, by which the wizard often destroyed by instant death a person or an entire family that he did not like—the wizard it was said being seen at twilight only of an evening flying about to do mischief—whenever such a person was found, I say, it was not for him to exculpate himself. He was seized by a mob, tied to a tree with ropes, and lightwood piled around him and set on fire and he burned to death with as little compunction or remorse of conscience as, in the Roman inquisition, many of the most enlightened and well disposed to peace and good order, were brought to a fiery ordeal for the common good." [14]

Hitchcock learned that witches and wizards "can take the form of owls and fly about at night and at day return home in the form of women and men; that they can take the heart and the spirit out of living men and cause their death; that they can cripple people by shooting rags or blood into their legs through a reed or out of their mouths." "Formerly," he was told, "the Indians have been known to knock old women regarded as witches on the head and throw them into the water. Now there is a law against it, but even last year an old woman was killed as a witch." [15]

Adair says that "there are not greater bigots in Europe, nor persons more superstitious, than the Indians, (especially the women) concerning the power of witches, wizards, and evil spirits. It is the chief feature of their idle winter night's chat: and both they, and several of our traders, report very incredible and shocking stories. They will affirm that they have seen, and distinctly, most surprising apparitions, and heard horrid shrieking noises." [16]

Suspicion of witchcraft attached not only to doctors and graduates but to old persons of both sexes. I was told that formerly the Creeks did not allow their children to hang around where old people were conversing, for they thought that by standing around them and looking at them they would get into the habit of telling lies and also that

---

[14] Stiggins, Ms.   [15] Hitchcock, Ms. notes.   [16] Adair, Hist. Am. Inds., p. 36.

the old people might bewitch them. This does not speak very highly for the reputation for veracity enjoyed by the aged. It was thought that any old man who had passed through as many fastings as most of them had undergone at that time of life might be a wizard. It was feared that he might shoot a pain into the child or injure it in some other manner. One of my informants said he had often been slapped hard enough to be knocked down when he was standing near some of the old people. The following from Adair gives additional information regarding witchcraft among the Chickasaw, and contains the only extant account of an exorcism to preserve the house from evil influences. He says:

"In the year 1765, an old physician, or prophet, almost drunk with spirituous liquors, came to pay me a friendly visit: his situation made him more communicative than he would have been if quite sober. When he came to the door, he bowed himself half bent, with his arms extended north and south, continuing so perhaps for the space of a minute. Then raising himself erect, with his arms in the same position, he looked in a wild frightful manner, from the south-west toward the north, and sung on a low bass key *Yo Yo Yo Yo*, almost a minute, then *He He He He*, for perhaps the same space of time, and *Wa Wa Wa Wa*, in like manner; and then transposed and accented those sacred notes several different ways, in a most rapid guttural manner. Now and then he looked upwards, with his head considerably bent backward; his song continued about a quarter of an hour. As my door which was then opened stood east, his face of course looked toward the west; but whether the natives thus usually invoke the deity, I cannot determine; yet as all their winter houses have their doors toward the east, had he used the like solemn invocations there, his face would have consequently looked the same way, contrary to the usage of the heathens. After his song, he stepped in: I saluted him, saying, 'Are you come my beloved old friend?' he replied, *Arahre-O*, 'I am come in the name of Oea.'[16a] I told him, I was glad to see, that in this mad age, he still retained the old Chikkasah virtues. He said, that as he came with a glad heart to see me his old friend, he imagined he could not do me a more kind service, than to secure my house from the power of the evil spirits of the north, south, and west,—and, from witches, and wizards, who go about in dark nights, in the shape of bears, hogs, and wolves, to spoil people: 'the very month before, added he, we killed an old witch, for having used destructive charms.' Because a child was suddenly taken ill, and died, on the physician's false evidence, the father went to the poor helpless old woman who was sitting innocent,

---

[16a] This is **álali**, "I come," followed by a simple exclamation. The being "Oea" is contributed by Adair's imagination.

and unsuspecting, and sunk his tomahawk into her head, without the least fear of being called to an account. They call witches and wizards, *Ishtabe*, and *Hoollabe*, 'man-killers,' and 'spoilers of things sacred.'[17]

"My prophetic friend desired me to think myself secure from those dangerous enemies of darkness, for (said he) *Tarooa Ishtohoollo-Antarooare*, 'I have sung the song of the great holy one.'[18] The Indians are so tenacious of concealing their religious mysteries, that I never before observed such an invocation on the like occasion— adjuring evil spirits, witches, etc. by the awful name of the deity."[19]

This exorcism probably gives a clue to one of the reasons why the doors of the winter houses opened eastward; also the reason for the eastward orientation of most of the chiefs' houses in the square ground.

From the Texas Alabama I learned that a witch operated by taking a small raveling of wool which he talked to and blew upon and then sent through the air to the person he wished to injure. It would go into this person and prevent him from breathing, or hurt him in some other way, so as to endanger his life unless the trouble were located. If a doctor were called in he would take a sharp bit of glass, make some incisions over the place where the raveling had lodged, and, applying a horn to the spot, suck the foreign body out. These bodies looked black, red, or blue. My informant had seen the operation performed and the bodies that were removed. Besides woolen ravelings, ravelings of other kinds might be used, charcoal, and probably bones also. The injuries inflicted by charcoal were very serious.

Sometimes a man or woman who disliked a hunter would make medicine in order to keep him from killing game. The Alabama called this impiafōtcī, "to make him kill nothing."[19a] The hunter might go to a doctor, however, and have him make medicine to counteract that of the witch. A man once saw an eagle catching fish and used the impiafōtcī against it so that it could get nothing and almost starved to death. The eagle went out in all directions and caught nothing, but finally he went up into the sky and caught a fish there. Next day the same thing happened and now the man who had tried to bewitch the eagle began to get thin, and finally he died. The eagle had beaten him.

From the same source I learned that a man who had acquired the black art would sometimes wake up in the morning and see a hatchet or a knife on his breast. Then, when he killed someone by means of

[17] Ishto, big; abi, to kill; holo, what is sacred; abi, to kill.
[18] Taloa, song; ishto, big; holo, sacred; ontaloali, or intaloali, I have sung to them.
[19] Adair, Hist. Am. Inds., pp. 176-177.
[19a] Piafo signifies "unlucky"; impiafōtcī, "to cause one to be unlucky."

his arts, he was sure to be found out and killed himself by the man's relatives with the same kind of weapon he had seen in his vision.

In speaking of doctors I have mentioned the native belief that they owed their power to animals of various kinds, but that if these became too strong they would kill the doctor and leave him. The same idea appears in witchcraft, although my information here is specifically from the Alabama and Koasati. When a man became a witch these Indians believed he was full of lizards, which compelled the person of whom they had possession to kill someone every little while. If he did not they would begin to bite him and would finally devour him. Such a person could be cured, however, by undergoing a treatment to expel the lizards.

After a would-be wizard had completed his course of training, the teacher directed him to begin by killing one of his own family. He gave him medicine and told him to go and do so immediately. If he said he would not kill his own people, the instructor answered "Go on! you said that is what you wanted to do." But if he urged him repeatedly to no purpose, he said, "All right! kill a fox squirrel and bring it here!" After he had done so, the instructor said, "Throw it on top of the house." The wizard-novice did this, and after the body had remained so long that it stank, the other said, "Eat it!" Then the instructor conducted him to a place where there was water and said, "Vomit on the water." So he threw up and discharged lizards until the water was covered. The witching powers went with them.

The Koasati cured a wizard by binding spunk wood all over his chest and belly, taking him to a place where there was water, and rolling him over and over there, when he would throw up lizards in the manner described.

A milder form of witchcraft was that exercised by a man or woman to inspire love in a person of the opposite sex. The following account of such a conjuration is also from the Alabama of Texas.

When a youth fell in love he would sometimes, especially if he were rejected, go to a male or female conjurer for assistance. Then the conjurer would take some tobacco, put it into a small deerskin sack, sing, and repeat the girl's name, and blow into it through a short cane. After doing this four times he would wrap it up in a handkerchief and give it to the young man. The latter would then put on his head band and his other fine clothing, sprinkle some tobacco over his clothes, make a cigarette, and blow the smoke all over himself. Then the girl would fall in love with him. A girl could make a man fall in love with her in precisely the same way. Sometimes, however, this would be tried in vain several times. Then the conjurer would go to a small brook and make a little water hole, perhaps half a foot deep. He would blow into this four times through a cane, repeating the girl's name each time. The youth would then come there, stoop down and drink some of the water, and throw it up again into the pool. He would do this four times. Then he would divide the dam that held the water in this pool and let it all run away. After that he would go to a large creek, remove his clothing, and dive under water four times. Then he would come out and lie in the bushes almost all day (having started out early in the morning) so that no one could see him. About 3 o'clock he started home, avoiding meeting or speaking to anyone. In perhaps a week he would dress himself up as before and go to see the girl he was in love with, who would then fall in love with him. Sometimes, however, the girl's mother would make medicine against him so that he could not succeed in spite of all his efforts.

DISEASES AND REMEDIES

GENERAL REMARKS

To the discussion of this subject I will prefix the following general remarks from Bartram regarding the diseases of the Indians in his time. However superficial, it has the advantage of being the only statement of the kind belonging to an early period from a man competent to express anything like a scientific opinion.

"The Indians seem in general healthier than the whites, have fewer diseases, and those they have not so acute or contagious as those amongst us.

"The small-pox sometimes visits them, and is the most dreaded of all diseases.

"Dysentery, pleurisy, intermittent fevers, epilepsy and asthma, they have at times.

"The hooping-cough is fatal among their children, and worms very frequent. . . .

"They have the venereal disease amongst them in some of its stages; but by their continence, temperance, powerful remedies, skill in applying them, and care, it is a disease which may be said to be uncommon. In some towns it is scarcely known, and in none rises to that state of virulency which we call a *pox*, unless sometimes amongst the white traders who themselves say, as well as the Indians, that it might be eradicated if the traders did not carry it with them to the nations when they return with their merchandise; these contract the disorder before they set off, and it generally becomes virulent by the time they arrive, when they apply to the Indian doctors to get cured." [20]

We will now turn to the native conception of diseases and their remedies. This is best illustrated in the abstract by the following myth collected by Dr. Frank Speck from an old Creek medicine man known as Kabitcimala (Kapitca imala), or Laslie Cloud.

---

[20] Bartram, Trans. Am. Eth. Soc., vol. III, pp. 43–44.

"The old people, our Maskogi ancestors, were gathered together in the olden times. The deer said that he was the cause of a sickness. So he made the medicine for its cure. The panther said that he was the cause of one. It was he, then, who made the medicine for that trouble. Then again, the bear was the cause of one. He said that he made the medicine for that. Then the snake caused one, and made its medicine. Then again, the hog said he was the cause of one, and he made the medicine for it. The bird was the cause of one, and he made the medicine for it. Then again, the wildcat was the cause of one, and he made the medicine for it. Then again, the horse said that he was the cause of one, and he made the medicine for it. Then the beaver said he was the cause of one, and made the medicine for it. Then again, the dog said he was the cause of one, and made the medicine for it. Then again, the otter said he was the cause of one, and made the medicine for it. Then again, the fish said it was the cause of one, and made the medicine for it. Then again, the game animals said they were the cause of one, and made the medicine for it. Then again, the water animals said they were the cause of one, and made the medicine for it. Then again, the animals of the sea-shore said they were the cause of one, and made the medicine for it. Then again, the animals in the sea said they were the cause of one, and made the medicine for it. Then the snake tribe said they were causes and made medicines for them. Then again, the animals-moving-about-in-the-water said they were causes and made medicines for them. Then the small-living-things-in-the-water said they were causes and made medicines for them. Then again, the raccoon said he was the cause of one and made the medicine for it. Then the white-hog (opossum) said he was the cause of one and made the medicine for it. Then again, the sky-hog said he was the cause of one and made medicine for it. Then again, the rainbow said he was the cause of one and made the medicine for it. Then again, the spirits of the dead said they were causes and made medicines for them. Then again, the different kinds of dirt said they were causes and made medicines for them. Then again, new-fire-when-it-is-cold said it was the cause of one and made the medicine for it. Then again, the buzzard said he was the cause of one and made the medicine for it. Then again, living-people said they were causes and made medicines for them. Then again, the turkey said he was the cause of one and made the medicine for it. Then again, the wolf-in-the-water said he was the cause of one and made the medicine for it. Then again, the land-wolf said he was the cause of one and made the medicine for it. Then again, the rattlesnake said he was the cause of one and made the medicine for it. Then again, the owl said he was the cause of one and made the medicine for it. Then again, what-is-inside-of-me said he was the cause of one and made the medicine for it."[20a]

Mooney's Cherokee version of the "Origin of Disease and Medicine"[21] agrees with the above in tracing diseases to the animals, but according to this the animals created diseases in self-defence, and the plant creation volunteered the remedies which were to counteract them. The two stories agree, however, in tracing diseases mainly to the animals. This my Natchez informant also confirmed.

Long as is the list given by Speck's informant it by no means exhausts the alleged sources of disease and it is difficult to see how some of these could have prescribed their own cures. The myth does not perhaps represent the philosophical idea held by all doctors but it is universally true of the Creeks that animals along with many other things were supposed to occasion diseases, that there were cures for each, and that the remedies used often had some kind of resemblance, real or supposed, to the reputed causes. We will take up these causes of disease in order with the information which I have obtained regarding the method of treating each malady. The greater part of this information was obtained from Jackson Lewis, to which I have added a small amount from various other Indians and what could be gleaned from earlier writings.

The same evolution which had carried the Creeks to a point where they had schools of medicine, even though rudimentary in their nature, had brought about specialization both in the medicines used and in the practice of the different physicians. I have already spoken of the separate class of kīłas or diagnosticians and the common or family doctors. Among regular practitioners, however, there was a further specialization. Each doctor did not pretend to cover the whole field of medicine. One would treat for the deer, one for the many snakes, one for the disorders contracted from graves, and so on. It was a common thing to specialize on diseases due to thunder. A doctor might tell what he knew of the disease but refer the patient to another if the method to be employed in treating it had not been given to him.

According to my Natchez informant one who had been struck by lightning and had afterwards recovered could cure diseases of all kinds.

The diseases were named from those animals or objects which the symptoms seemed to simulate or recall. Thus the water animals brought diseases of the stomach, bowels, liver, etc., the fish and snail (làbo), which exude slime like phlegm, caused diseases of the lungs, and so on. Sometimes the medicine contained only one thing, sometimes several. It would vary also with the class of creatures causing the trouble and the particular representative of that class.

[20a] Memoirs Am. Anth. Asso., vol. II, pt. 2, pp. 148–149.
[21] 19th Ann. Rept. Bur. Amer. Ethn., pt. I, pp. 250–252.

Thus the same basal medicines were used in curing diseases caused by water creatures, but diseases caused by particular water beings such as the water wolf, the rainbow, or the water tiger, would require some additions.   On the other hand we find single remedies employed in curing diseases due to the eye and tongue of the deer which are combined in the remedy for the deer disease.

CREEK MEDICINES

Deer diseases.—There was a disease produced by the common deer, one produced by "the many deer," a name used for all species and varieties of deer, and one produced by a newly born fawn or a fawn still in its mother's womb.   This last is called the "soft deer" (itco lowagi).   The eye of the deer will produce eye troubles and the tongue of the deer throat troubles.   The prescription for the common deer disease, the symptoms of which appear to be rheumatic pains in any part of the body, was to take some deer's potato (itco imaha), pāsa, itco hitcigu (a very fragrant weed looking something like goldenrod), cedar (atcīna), and a small piece of the tender end of the summer grapevine.   These were to be boiled together and the person steamed in them, more being taken internally.   As in all other cases to these ingredients must be added, in order to produce any results, the formula repeated by the doctor four times and blown into the medicine through a cane tube.   In treating "the many deer" and fawn diseases the same medicines were employed, only the formulæ being varied.   In treating the "deer eyes" disease itco hitcigu is used alone and in treating the "deer tongue" disease miko hoyanīdja. By other informants I was told that the common deer disease was rheumatism or neuralgia or sometimes a severe headache, and when it was incurable, or at least very acute, it was considered to be the "soft deer" disease (or "limber deer" disease—itco lowagi).

According to one of these men the "deer chief" disease (itco miko) was a name given to rheumatism when it was in one place, but evidently it was rheumatism of the severe type, for Jackson Lewis said that unless well treated it swelled the joints and sometimes lamed a man for life.   For it he used itco imaha and the bark scraped off of the wild crabapple (itco impàkana) in some quantity, a sprig of cedar, and four roots of the pāsa.   The swollen and inflamed places were steamed with this.

Tuggle has the following about this disease:

"Echo-polsa [itco pulsi]—Deer sickness.

"The medicine is made from the deer-potato or echo-mahhar [itco imaha], mixed in water.

"Song:

Hohtikee.
Hohtikee.

Hohtikee.
Echo.
Hohchetice.
Hohtikee.
Hohtikee.
Hohtikee.
Echo.
Mikkatee.

'Translation:

Hohtikee [hàtki], white.
Echo [itco], deer.
Hachetice [from hatci], tail.
Hotikee, white.
Echo, deer.
Mikkatee [mikati], has been king." [22]

According to Jackson Lewis, there is a grub which lives in the nostrils of the deer and comes out of them in the fall as a little butterfly called kauûlgi in Hitchiti and tcoànàga (itco hanako) in Muskogee. This is a good sign of the presence of deer and is sometimes found forming in deer. By the Indians it is considered to be the cause of catarrh. This belief was confirmed by Zachariah Cook. In treating it Jackson Lewis used the itco hitcigu and the itco imaha, with which might be included the pāsa. After these have been boiled in water and allowed to cool they are inhaled through the nostrils. He declared that he had cured numerous cases by means of this medicine.

The bear disease.—The patient is taken with a violent fever, accompanied by thirst for cold water, and he has frequent evacuations of the bowels. This trouble Jackson Lewis said was not very difficult to control. According to Zachariah Cook, this disease is called ponàtà haledji, which refers to the bear without naming him. The patient has a high fever and is out of his head; he is troubled about his mouth, pulls at the bed clothes, and gathers them in his arms as if he would pull them all together. One doctor told Cook that he could always cure this disease if he could get to the patient in time.[23]

The blood-of-the-bear disease.—The patient vomits up blood, or at least spits it up continually. The treatment is to take roots of the miko hoyanīdja, and roots of the frostweed (hitutape), mix these with water and give the decoction to the patient internally. If this does not appear to be as efficacious as desired, parings of the root of the kīstuwa, the "red root" of the whites, are put into a bottle along with cold water and some of this liquid drunk from time to time.

The bison disease.—I learned that there was such a disease but no facts regarding it.

[22] Ms., Bur. Amer. Ethn.
[23] See p. 644.

The rabbit disease.—The patient has pain in the lower part of the abdomen and is unable to pass water easily, what is passed being very red. The eyes are very yellow and there is sometimes paralysis in the lower parts of the body. Treatment: A bundle of stalks of a certain plant, for which I was unable to get either the native or English name, is procured, boiled in water, and administered. This plant is described as a grass or reed growing near streams to the height of 1½ or 2 feet, having leaves much resembling the leaves of the cane. The fruit is very thin and flutters from the stalk, which is jointed. Jackson Lewis was so enthusiastic about the medicinal properties of this plant that he declared it had been known to cure even those cases accompanied by paralysis of the lower limbs, and no formula was needed with it.

The raccoon disease.—This usually afflicts children; the patients are in poor health with greatly distended stomachs.

The squirrel disease.—The patient's gums are so inflamed that he can hardly eat. Treatment: A small quantity of bark of the red oak and hickory is taken from the places where the tree trunks enter the ground, boiled in water, and cooled, after which the patient rinses out his mouth with the infusion. He must also refrain from eating anything that is very soft.

The dog disease.—There are severe pains in the bowels and stomach accompanied by vomiting.[24] Treatment: Use parings of sassafras roots, adding to them a small handful of a fine grass known to the Indians as "dog's bed." These are boiled in water and a little given to the patient to drink warm. In repeating the formula for this disease the points of the compass are successively addressed but no colors are mentioned.

Tuggle has the following to say about the dog disease:

"Cramps in the stomach, or dog-sickness, is caused by a dog.

"The medicine is prepared from tobacco, cut up and put in water, making a weak tea, which the patient drinks and also uses as a wash.

"The song is sung while blowing in the water, in order to properly medicate the preparation. Each stanza is repeated four times and after each the doctor blows into the medicine. Finally both stanzas are sung four times and blowing done between.

> Yoh-ho-lee
> Yoh-ho-lee
> Yoh-ho-lee
> Efa
> Polsa
> Thlohko
> Elahtee
> Hahlahtee
>   St Chay

---

[24] According to Hitchcock, Megillis Hadjo, a famous Tukabachee Kila living in 1842, also identified the dog disease with pains in the bowels.

Hoh-loh-tee
Hoh-loh-tee
Hoh-loh-tee
    St Chay

"Translation:

Yohholee [yulihĭ], be easy
Efa [ifa], dog
Polsa [pulsĭ], sickness
Thlahkko [lăko], large
Elathe [ilitá], dead
Hohlahtee [hálati, to hold, to pull?], cramping
St Chay [tcē], stop, or like *Selah.*   It merely indicates the end of a sentence, or an idea.

"In the second verse—

Hohlohtee [hálati], holding him, or, it's got him." [25]

The wolf disease.—The symptoms and treatment are the same as for the dog disease.[26]   But see below.

The rat or mouse disease.—The only information I have regarding a disease caused by rats or mice is the following from the Tuggle manuscript.   It will be seen that it may have been only the wolf disease under another name:

"The medicine for pains in the temple (headache) is mikko-whe-ar-ne-chah [miko hoyanĭdja], or red-root.

"It is put in water and during the chant or song the medicine man blows in the water through a cane and after the song is complete, each verse being sung four times and then the entire song four times, the water is poured over the patient's head.   This is repeated four days, always before eating in the morning.

"This sickness is caused by rats or mice, and the song is to drive them away.   Some say Yaha, the Wolf, causes it.   It is sung in a low monotonous tone—a chant.   Each verse is repeated four times and after each repetition the doctor blows into the medicine.

Hah-noh-noh-hee
Hah-noh-noh-hee
Hah-noh-noh-hee
Chaysee chah-tee
Holochee chah-tee
Man-kaht-kan
    Hah-yeen
Yah-fee noh-hokee

Hah-noh-noh-hee
Hah-noh-noh-hee
Hah-noh-noh-hee
Chaysee lahnee
Holochee lahnee

---

[25] Ms., Bur. Amer. Ethn
[26] Megillis Hadjo attributed "stricture in the bladder" to obsession by a mad wolf.

Mankaht kan
Hahyeen
Yah-fee noh-hokee

Hoh-noh-noh-hee!
Hoh-noh-noh-hee!
Hoh-noh-noh-hee!
Chaysee lustee
Holochee lustee
Man kohtkan
Hohyeen
Yohfeenohhokee

Hoh-noh-noh-hee
Hoh-noh-noh-hee
Hoh-noh-noh-hee
Chaysee hutkee
Holochee hutkee
Maukabbkan
Hahyeen
Yohfee nohhokee

"The translation of this song is as follows:

Hohnohnohhee, gallop slowly away (like a rat galloping)
Chaysee [tcisi], rat or mouse
Chahtee [tcati], red
Holochee [aholotci], cloud
Mauhobt can [? (tcaka, my head)], my head
Hohyeen [haihoyin], hot
Yoh fee noh-ho-kee [finōki, shaking?], roaring

"Literally:

Gallop away
Gallop away
Gallop away
Red rat
Red cloud
My head
Is hot
Is roaring

"The 'Red cloud' may refer to a rush of blood to the head.

"In the second verse the color of the rat is changed to 'lohnee' [lāni], yellow, and so with the cloud.

"In the third verse the rat is 'lustee' [låsti], black, and also the cloud.

"In the fourth verse the rat is 'white' [håtki], as is also the cloud."

The lion disease (Lion = "Person-eater," Isti-papa).—According to Jackson Lewis the symptoms of this are a kind of cramp or "holding" inside of the chest. According to Zachariah Cook this disease is cholera morbus. Jackson Lewis said he had never treated it but Cook said it was cured by using the "big medicine" (hilis låkåt), which is the "butterfly plant." The song used with this refers to the myths telling how Rabbit left the Lion on the other side of the ocean. Cook had learned of this largely through a virulent epidemic of cholera near 1870–1875.

The wildcat and panther diseases.—According to Cook powerful cramps in the stomach are attributed to a wildcat or some such powerful animal, but, beyond this and the reference by Speck, I have no information regarding a wildcat or panther disease.

The mole disease (táko aledji).—The symptoms are cramps in the bowels, colic, etc. This information was from Zachariah Cook, who did not know how it was treated.

The opossum disease.—According to Zachariah Cook this was the name given to croup (nukłahe) in children. Jackson Lewis did not know the native explanation for this trouble.

The *beaver* (itchaswa), *otter* (osána), and *muskrat* (oktcûtko) are supposed to bring about liver complaint, bowel troubles, gravel, etc., like some of the other water animals. Megillis Hadjo, the Tukabahchee kiła mentioned by Hitchcock, held that "costiveness proceeds from two beavers in the bowels of the patient, who have made a dam in him; if pains are added, a bear is inside fighting with the beavers." This agrees with what I was told by William McCombs to the effect that cramps in the bowels were due to the beaver and badger, the beaver because he dams up streams as the bowels are stopped up and the badger because he is thought to have bellyache all the time and the continual running off of the bowels is thought to be due to him. The treatment is much like that used with diseases caused by the other water animals, but I have no specific information regarding it. The prescription contains some of the same remedies as those used in diseases due to water snakes and turtles and some that are different.

The eagle disease.—The patient has cramps in the muscles of the neck or a "crick in the neck" so that the head is turned to one side and can not be moved back. Jackson Lewis said it was probably due to the fact that the patient had handled an eagle feather. According to Mr. McCombs it was believed that the eagle caused the trouble by perching on the back of the neck and must be driven off by the fumes of cedar.

The buzzard disease.—When a child vomits and purges a great deal he is afflicted by the buzzard.

The many-snakes disease.—The "many snakes" have already been mentioned as a term used to include all sorts of serpents and lizards, real and imaginary, though not frogs, toads, or alligators. They are the active causes of a great many diseases such as swellings, abscesses, etc.

The gatherers-in-the-waters disease.—This term is used for the inhabitants of the water elsewhere described. The person suffering from this disease has pains in the stomach or bowels, more often the latter, and retches and vomits at times. Sometimes he also has pains in the sides and back. In treating, the roots of a sycamore—the sycamore being a water tree—willow roots, a bunch of small roots from the birch, a piece of wood broken from a stick lying in shallow water in the woods and nearly rotted, are collected. With them is put some water dipped out of a small whirlpool in running water, and a little water from a hairlike line often seen on ponded water just back of a little fall. Then more water is added, the whole boiled and used warm, a little being drunk, some put on the body, and some used in steaming the body.

Regarding the "snake disease" Zachariah Cook said that the name was given to swellings, boils, carbuncles arising in several places, and inflammatory rheumatism. Certain rheumatic pains or certain kinds of paralysis were attributed to the "unseen-snakes-in-the-water disease" (ayá haigida), or "many-animals-of-the-water disease" (wiak wilagi sûlgat). This last is evidently the "many-snakes disease." It seems that these creatures taken separately could produce diseases also. According to Cook the water tiger (wi-katca) causes congestion of the stomach, the water-king deer (wīofûts miko) something similar to rheumatism of the bowels, and the water buffalo (wī yanasa) an inward corruption of the liver something like the snake disease.

The snake disease.—By this is meant simply snake bite. The medicinal plant used by Jackson Lewis blooms about July and the flower is white. When ready to open it shows a number of teeth inside just like the teeth of a snake. The roots are said to be large and oval. One of my informants was treated by a doctor in a case of snake bite. The doctor chewed up some of this root and then sucked the wound.

The snake medicine, of which a specimen was furnished by Caley Proctor, and which may be identical with the above, was *Manfreda virginica*, called abi-tcápko ("long stem") in Creek. It was said to be a sure cure both for snake bite and the bite of a centipede. The roots were boiled in water and the bite washed with the liquid. Another way employed by a doctor was to take some common tobacco into his mouth, suck the bite four times and as he did so hum four times the following formula: tohiudjidī tohiłákodi solonk, the words of which seem to have no meaning.

When this snake medicine was not to be had the summer grape (pálko łáko, "big grape") might be substituted. The tendrils and soft, succulent ends of the vines were boiled thoroughly and the infusion afterward given to the patient to drink.

Some doctors attained such proficiency that they were not afraid to pick up any kind of snake. A man named Keeka, living between

Beggs and Hamilton, possessed this power and he would not allow any of his family to kill a snake. Upon one occasion Adair "saw the Chikkasah Archi-magus chew some snake-root, blow it on his hands, and then take up a rattlesnake without damage." In another place he has the following to say about native snake medicines:

"I do not remember to have seen or heard of an Indian dying by the bite of a snake, when out at war, or a hunting; although they are often bitten by the most dangerous snakes—everyone carries in his shot-pouch, a piece of the best snake-root, such as the *Seneeka*, or fern-snake-root,—or the wild hore-hound, wild plantain, St. Andrew's cross, and a variety of other herbs and roots, which are plenty, and well known to those who range the American woods, and are exposed to such dangers, and will effect a thorough and speedy cure if timely applied. When an Indian perceives he is struck by a snake, he immediately chews some of the root, and having swallowed a sufficient quantity of it, he applies some to the wound; which he repeats as occasion requires, and in proportion to the poison the snake has infused into the wound. For a short space of time, there is a terrible conflict through all the body, by the jarring qualities of the burning poison, and the strong antidote; but the poison is soon repelled through the same channels it entered, and the patient is cured." [27]

I do not know whether the following formula was used in cases of snake bite or a more esoteric kind of snake sickness. It is from the Tuggle collection.

"After preparing this medicine [for "snake sickness"], the medicine-man sang this song:

> O, spirit of the white fox, come
> O, spirit of the white fox, come
> O, spirit of the white fox, come
> O, hater of snakes, come
> Snakes [who] have hurt this man, come
> Come, O white fox, and kill this snake.
>
> O, spirit of the red fox, come, etc.
>
> O, spirit of the black fox, come, etc.[28]

James Islands and N. L. Alexander, two Creek Indians, told General Hitchcock that "a case of salivation . . . was caused by two rattlesnakes in the mouth," adding that "they required five dollars for a prescription." This disease is evidently different from all of those snake diseases above mentioned, except possibly the last.

The turtle disease.—The symptom of this is a chronic cough which results in appreciably reducing the flesh of the victim. Treatment:

---

[27] Adair, Hist. Am. Inds., pp. 235–236.

[28] Ms., Bur. Amer. Ethn. Probably one verse, referring to a blue or yellow fox, has been lost. This formula is peculiar in beginning with the east, but it is impossible to tell whether the points of the compass are taken in sinistral order or in dextral order.

Make an infusion in water of the roots of a plant called "turtle's liver" (lutca logi). This is not found in the Creek Nation but in the country of the Cherokee (Oklahoma), and it has small circular leaves and beautiful blue flowers. If it can not be obtained, substitute for it a small piece of buckeye and a small piece of devil's shoestring. The patient must drink small quantities of this decoction from time to time warm. Warm cloths máy also be put into it and then around the throat and chest.

Zachariah Cook, however, gave the name "turtle disease" (hilutca) to a hard boil forming one head. He mentioned another disease called "turtles-of-the-water" or "many turtles" (lutca sulgat), which is some sort of stomach trouble or liver complaint. It is almost identical with a disease known as "wolf-of-the-water" (wiofi yaha), and the two are treated alike, but I did not learn how.

The terrapin (lutca lobotski) disease.—According to Zachariah Cook this deforms a person by cramping his stomach or raising a lump on his shoulder. It is said that small people were affected in this way, and this suggests that it may be a name applied to the disease producing hunchbacks. In the song used in treating this disease the terrapin is called lutca hayegi, "the turtle rattles are made of."

The alligator was not accused, so far as Jackson Lewis could remember, of causing any disease, but Zachariah Cook said that it was included in the turtle disease, by which I suppose he meant that it was an animal which produced the same trouble either separately or in conjunction with the turtle.

The perch disease (sándálákwá, perch).—The symptoms of this are a very acute attack of coughing which the patient can hardly stop. Treatment: Sassafras and the devil's shoestring are boiled and about a tablespoonful given at a dose.

The "periwinkle" disease.—Tuggle has the following to say about this:

'Karpochee, or Periwinkle sickness, caused by the periwinkle. The jaws swell as in mumps.

" The medicine is prepared from the gourd, Phibbee [fibí], either from the green leaves, or from the seed, when the leaves can not be obtained. In the following song which goes with this medicine each verse is repeated four times and after each time the medicine is blown into as is customary in other cases. At the end the entire song is repeated four times, and the blowings again take place.

" The song:

Che-kee
Che-kee
Thlah-kotee
Che-kee
Che-kee
Che-kee

Thlah-kotee
Che-kee
Che-kee
Che-kee
Thlah-kotee

Che-kee
Che-ko-chetee
Che-kee
Che-ko-chetee
Che-kee
Che-ko-chetee
Foh-yoh-yoke
Thlah-kotee
Foh-yoh-yoke
Thlah-kotee
Foh-yoh-yoke
Thlah-kotee

"Meaning of words:

Cheke [tcikhĭ], rough (up and down) [raised in mounds]
Thlahkotee [łăkotĭ], big (large, swollen)
Chekochetee [tcutkutcitĭ], little
Fohyohyoke [from folotki], twisted

"Literal translation:

Rough, rough, big
Rough, rough, big
Rough, rough, big

Rough, rough, little
Rough, rough, little
Rough, rough, little

Twisted big
Twisted big
Twisted big" [29]

Unless there is some usage of the word periwinkle other than that known to me, as applied to a small marine shell, it would seem as if Tuggle must have erred in translating the name of this disease. For a long period of time the periwinkle can have played no part in the life of the Creek Indians.

The slug disease.—The patient has some cough but more particularly a very considerable expectoration of phlegm. Treatment: The same as for the perch disease but with a different formula.

The millepede disease.—The patient coughs and is so hoarse as almost to lose his voice. Treatment: An infusion of ginseng is to be drunk very warm.

The ant disease (tákodja', ant).—According to Zachariah Cook when matter runs from a boil leaving holes the trouble is attributed to the ant.

---

[29] Ms., Bur. Amer. Ethn.

The *"mastodon" disease.*—It was asserted by William McCombs that there was such a disease recognized, its native name being Laktaga, "the greatest of great [animals]." This name may perhaps have been applied to some mythic animal on the basis of mastodon or other bones found from time to time.

The *hàtckutcàp disease.*—This is caused by a mythical animal described elsewhere.[29a] Those who happen to see this creature have a severe fever and some have been known to die.

The *hàtcko-fàski disease.*—This is produced by another mythical animal described elsewhere. I have no information regarding the malady itself.[29a]

The *good-snake disease.*—A disease is produced by the bodyless celestial snake described in the section on religion.[29b] In treating it Jackson Lewis took roots of the sycamore, willow, and birch, sprigs of cedar, and seed pods of the red sumac which he boiled in water, using the resulting liquid to give the patient a sweat bath. A little was also given the patient to drink. The treatment was repeated on several successive days.

The *rainbow disease.*—As its name implies, this was supposed to be caused by the rainbow. Its symptoms are like those of the preceding and it was treated similarly.

The little people and giants have elsewhere been described, as also the effects produced by them in bewildering persons and leading them astray.[29c] The disease caused by them is known as labàtkàdilõga, "gathered on land"—i. e., not in the water—or "outside gathering on land."[29d] Treatment: Procure four little forked limbs of the post oak, one little sprig of the wild plum—a sprig of the huckleberry (tsafàknà), one of the mistletoe, one of the red haw, one of the cedar and one of a bush like the huckleberry but growing 4 feet high and bearing in June. The red haw and cedar are taken because the giants are said to feed upon their berries. To these things is added a pine cone if it can be gotten, if not a sprig of pine with the needles on; also a sprig of the winter huckleberry (owīsa); a kind of highbush huckleberry which ripens in November and during the winter, and grows on rough ground far up in the mountains; a sprig of the black haw (silāwa); a sprig of the summer grape or "big grape"; a sprig of the winter grape or "little grape"; a sprig of the muscadine (tsoloswa); four sprigs from blackberry bushes; four sprigs from dewberry vines; one sprig from the raspberry; and finally sprigs of two plants which appear to be a large and a small variety of straw-

---

[29a] See p. 497.
[29b] See p. 494.
[29c] See pp. 496–497.
[29d] The word is compounded of labàtki, "straight," and adilõga, "together."

berry. Four shoots of each are taken. To all these may be added a
very small quantity of horsemint. The patient is to drink some of
this, sponge his body with the liquid, and use it in sweat bathing.
The doctor, as usual, sings over it and blows into it with a cane,
after which it is boiled and used warm. When the patient has recovered the doctor strictly enjoins him from using intoxicating drinks.

Zachariah Cook called this particular disease pneumonia, and said
that hitci påkpågi was put into the medicine as a "foundation."
When it had been compounded and conjured they sprinkled it about
around the house—four times around the outside and four times
around the inside alternately, i. e., once outside, then once inside,
and so until they were through. This was done for four successive
days by some one in the family selected for the purpose, after the
doctor had come and conjured the medicine, at about sunset.

The spirit-of-war disease.—When a person is not sick in bed but
keeps talking deliriously about war, battle, and things connected
with them, saying "there come the enemy" and using other similar
expressions until his health is injured and he is in danger of dying,
it is said that he is afflicted by the spirit of war. Treatment: Cut
four little forks from a post oak, take a quantity of horsemint, either
dead or fresh, a sprig of pine with the leaves on, and a quantity of
spicewood. Boil these in water, steam the patient with the infusion,
and when it is cold bathe him in it.

Thunder disease.—The symptoms of this were severe pains in the
head and arms. Sometimes the lightning shocks a person, almost
kills him, and makes him delirious. Treatment: Take a piece of
the "rattan vine," a sassafras root, and some gunpowder, and add
water to them. The "rattan vine" grows in the bottoms and is
called in Creek itō yektså, "strong wood." It does not grow thickly
anywhere. The mixture above described is not heated, but the
doctor repeats formulæ over it and blows into it through a tube 5
or 6 feet long, whereas the tube commonly used is only about 3 feet
long. The making of medicine for this disease is looked upon as
very important and nothing about it must be done triflingly. There
are doctors who are specialists in it.

The sun disease.—The patient has a sensation of heat in the crown
of the head, accompanied by general aching, and toward midday
falls about and becomes light headed. This trouble is caused by
the sun assisted by the morning star, the moon, and a certain red
star, and the disease is sometimes called a-i'lå. Treatment: Use
miko hoyanīdja, a piece of the root of the wild or domesticated sun-
flower, a puffball, and some angelica obtained from a drug store.
Mix these up with water and pour the whole cold over the head of
the patient, allowing it to run back into the dish from which it is
dipped. If this is repeated often the patient will almost surely
recover.

The fire disease.—Naturally enough fevers are often supposed to be occasioned by the fire, but there are several different kinds of fire responsible for them. According to one informant there are the new busk-ground fire (totkà mutcàsà), the hunters' fire, i. e., the fire which the hunters use while they are out (ponàtà hoboya imitotka), the fire the hunters build after they get home (totkà nàtkàbofa), and "the different kinds of fires" (also called totkà nàtkàbofa). According to Adair the old year's fire was considered "a most dangerous pollution."[30]

Diseases might also come from the paddle used in the stomp dance, and the other stomp dance accessories, as also from the unseen animals of the square ground.

Tuggle notes that according to some "all disease . . . is caused by the winds, which are born in the air and then descend to the earth."[31] By this he evidently means that the diseases are born in the air, not the winds. While it is often said that "sickness comes in the wind" it would seem that this applied rather to certain kinds of sickness caused by the winds, just as sickness was caused by the thunder, sun, etc., not that all sickness was so caused. This would perhaps account for the Chickasaw aversion to the north wind which, according to Adair, they called "very evil and accursed,"[30] though its origin in the cold quarter is sufficient explanation.

Disease was supposed to emanate from women during their monthly periods and attack men, especially in the spring of the year. This might be from contact with them or be brought by the wind blowing from them. According to Jackson Lewis the symptoms were a numbness, especially of the lower limbs, accompanied by nosebleed and headache, and a mental depression so great that the patient does not care whether he lives or dies. This agrees to some extent with Zachariah Cook's description of it as a kind of biliousness. A woman's period is called ibōski and the treatment for it ibōskilīlī. Both informants agreed that the medicine for it was miko hoyanīdja, which a man could drink, bathe in, and sweat-bathe in. Jackson Lewis said that the doctor sometimes took his patient away from the settlement, had him fast and then gave him the medicine and had him vomit. This treatment was sure to restore him perfectly.

Another dangerous source of disease was a dead body. This disease was called ikàn odjàlgi, which means "land owners," the dead being so called. Certain maleficent influences were believed to emanate from a dead body even after it was laid away in the ground, and persons in the vicinity were subject to aches and pains about

---

[30] Adair, Hist. Am. Inds., p. 22.　　　[31] Ms., Bur. Amer. Ethn.

the joints of the legs, and in other places. The ghost of the dead man was supposed to be the efficient cause of this. Even the dirt that fell upon one's clothing in digging a grave or covering up the body, or the dirt from a grave upon which one stepped, was apt to bring on this disorder. If one engaged in digging a grave he was likely to have pains in the back. Sometimes he had a chilly feeling across his back with pains running round to the front of his body and fatigue in all of the lower limbs. A person who dug a grave could also communicate the disease and this was the principal reason for the regulations to which he was subjected, and which are elsewhere described.[32] This disease would seem to have been some form of rheumatism—Tuggle calls it "pains in the knees or rheumatism"— but one informant described it as dropsy, or at all events ascribed such an origin to dropsy. Treatment: Miko hoyanīdja and spice-wood (kápápaska) were boiled in water, conjured in the usual manner, and divided into two parts, one hot and one cold. Then the affected parts were treated with the hot and cold medicines alternately.

According to Tuggle's informant, however, "the medicine is made from Ihee-so [wīso]—sassafras root." He gives the following formula to accompany it:

Me-kah-kee
Thlah-kah-kete
E-leen
E-kah-nah
So-feets-kaht
Te-tah-ker

Estee
Wah-keets-kaht
Te-tah-ken
Oh-than-etaht
Te-tah-ken

Oewa
Ahk-lope-kaht
Te-tah-ken

Literally translated:

Mekahkee [mikági], kings
Thlahkah-kete [łákakiti], big
Eleen [ilīn], dead
Ekahnah [ikána], land
So feets kaht [sufītckat], dig it
Tetahker [titaki], ready
Este [isti], people
Wahkeets [wakēts], lay it down
Tetahkee [titaki], ready

[32] See pp. 388-398.

Oh thlan etoht [ohłanitat], cover it up
Tetahken [titakin], ready
Oewa [oīwa], water
Ahkłopekaht [akłopikat], wash it
Tetanken [titakin], ready

Or—

Great kings are dead
Be ready to dig the grave

Let the people bury them
Let them be ready to cover them

Let the water be ready for washing.[33]

This disease was connected with the whole question of ghosts and preventive measures and medicines against them. The Texas Alabama believed that if a person who had been by a grave came near one who was sick the latter would have fits. My informant claimed that upon one occasion a number of persons who had been near a grave came in where he was lying sick and sat down around him, whereupon he became deaf and acted as if he were out of his head. Such fits were thought to be caused by ghosts, and, to induce them to leave, the doctor would put cedar leaves into a pot over the fire without any water. As these leaves parched the smoke arising from them would fill the house. The ghost would like this and go away. Another Alabama medicine used against ghosts was the leaves of the sweet bay, which were made into a tea, drunk, and vomited up. This was done twice.

Among the Creeks generally hitci pȧkpȧgi was the sovereign deterrent for ghosts, though hilis hȧtki or ginseng was also used.

The Texas Alabama believe that if one's hands and feet are pierced by the "poison briar" he will not get well, but I did not hear of any doctoring in connection with this.

The same people also mention a disease called łefka, of the origin of which I am ignorant. It is produced by trying to lift a load beyond the person's real ability, causing perhaps a strained tendon. They treated it by tying about the affected part a briar much like the kanta, called in their language bȧkco oktcȧko, "blue briar." At the same time they sang and blew upon the place. A white man was once cured in this way by two Indian women, but when one of my informants tried that remedy himself upon another occasion it would not work because he did not know the proper foimulæ.

When a person exhibited a horror of other people and, if he found himself suddenly where there were many, always ran away, they said that his disease was due to people—i. e., he was suffering from witchcraft. Says Swan:

[33] Tuggle, Ms., Bur. Amer. Ethn.

"Stitches in the side, or small rheumatic pains, which are frequent with them [the Creeks], are often considered as the effect of some magic wound. They firmly believe that their Indian enemies have the power of shooting them as they lie asleep, at the distance of 500 miles. They often complain of having been shot by a Choctaw or Chickasaw from the midst of these nations, and send or go directly to the most cunning and eminent doctress for relief." [34] Male doctors prescribed for witchcraft equally with women.

Some other diseases and some different methods of treating the above are given by Doctor Speck, to whose paper (Mem. Am. Anthrop. Assn., vol. II, pt. 2, pp. 121–133) the reader is referred. Also cf. the same writer's Yuchi paper, Anthrop. Pubs. Univ. Mus., I, pp. 132–135.

Sickness was sometimes attributed to the absence of the soul from the body, and this was probably assigned as a principal cause of disease as well as a secondary cause. It was then the object of the doctor to induce it to come back. I have an Alabama story telling of such an occurrence. This is given by the same people as the specific cause of "slow fever." [34a]

Adair gives us in one invaluable paragraph an account of the origin and naming of a new disease. He says:

"In 1767, the Indians were struck with a disease, which they were unacquainted with before. It began with sharp pains in the head, at the lower part of each of the ears, and swelled the face and throat in a very extraordinary manner, and also the testicles. It continued about a fortnight, and in the like space of time went off gradually, without any dangerous consequence, or use of outward or inward remedies: they called it *Wahka Abeeka*, 'the cattle's distemper,' or sickness. Some of their young men had by stealth killed and eaten a few of the cattle which the traders had brought up, and they imagined they had thus polluted themselves, and were smitten in that strange manner, by having their heads, necks, etc., magnified like the same parts of a sick bull. They first concluded, either to kill all the cattle, or send them immediately off their land, to prevent the like mischief, or greater ills from befalling the beloved people— for their cunning old physicians or prophets would not undertake to cure them, in order to inflame the people to execute the former resolution; being jealous of encroachments, and afraid the cattle would spoil their open cornfields; upon which account, the traders arguments had no weight with these red Hebrew philosophers. But fortunately one of their head warriors had a few cattle soon presented to him, to keep off the wolf; and his reasoning proved so weighty, as to alter their resolution, and produce in them a contrary belief." [35]

---

[34] Schoolcraft, Ind. Tribes, vol. v, p. 271.
[34a] See p. 666.
[35] Adair, Hist. Am. Inds., p. 132.

Besides the accounts of diseases and their cures already given I have considerable information regarding medicine plants and their uses in diseases for which I have no native explanation, although in some cases the name of the plant probably contains the supposed cause of the disease. The greater number of these were obtained from Jackson Lewis, another portion was from a Wīogufki Indian named Caley Proctor, a brother of the leader of the "Snake Indians," Eufaula Hadjo. He stated that he learned these things from an old Indian named Nokos īmała just before he died. To this I have added what I could learn among the Alabama of Texas, and some information from one of the few surviving Natchez Indians. The former varies somewhat from the rest on account of a difference in the Texas flora, while the latter has probably absorbed a great deal from the Cherokee among whom the surviving speakers of Natchez are living. A certain disorder was injected into Creek medical practice by the removal of the tribe west of the Mississippi, though Eakins's statement that "The roots and herbs they were accustomed to use in the '*old nation*' they have not yet been able to discover in their new country," must not be interpreted in a too sweeping manner.[36]

For the identification of the various plants I am indebted to Mr. Paul C. Standley, of the United States National Museum.

1. Miko hoyanīdja (a species of *Salix*, willow), "passer by of the chiefs," the medicine being supposed to pass by of its own power (G. W. G.) or perhaps "sovereign purgative." This is one of the two great busk medicines and as a remedy seems to have been thought more of than the pasa. It is known colloquially as the "red root," the roots of some being blood red and others pale red. Jackson Lewis said that it was used as part of the medicine in a great many complaints, such as fever with nausea and vomiting. According to Caley Proctor it was put in water and drunk by the patient, either cold or hot, in cases of internal fever, malaria, and biliousness. According to another informant it was used as "a graveyard medicine"— i. e., as he explained it, a medicine for dropsy—and also to cure the deer sickness. The patient was also bathed in it. It was used in conjunction with the spicewood (kȧpapȧskȧ) in cases of rheumatism and swellings. According to another informant the miko hoyanīdja and pasa together will cure "the clap" almost immediately. Eakins says simply that it was used in fevers.[36]

2. Pāsa. This is the "buttonsnake-root" of the whites, also sometimes called "bear grass," and its scientific name is *Eryngium yuccaefolium*. The Natchez called it awe'lwaih; the Koasati pase'. As above noted, it was the second of the two important busk medicines. Its use in conjunction with miko hoyanīdja has been mentioned. According to Caley Proctor, it was pounded up, mixed with water and drunk cold in cases of neuralgia and in kidney

36 Schoolcraft, Ind. Tribes, vol. I, p. 274.

troubles. It was also administered in cases of snake bite, and Jackson Lewis gave this as its principal use, in which he is confirmed by as old an authority as Adair.[37] Jackson Lewis added that it was used in conjunction with the "deer potato" in cases of rheumatism. Zachariah Cook said it was used for diseases of the spleen. According to another informant it was a great medicine to cleanse the system and purify the blood, and still another declared that its function at the busk was not so much to combat positive diseases as to produce a feeling of peace and tranquillity, an access of health as it were. Swan and other early writers, however, call this "the war physic." [38] Adair says "they frequently drink it to such excess as to impair their health, and sometimes so as to poison themselves by its acrid quality." [39] The Alabama and Koasati swallowed small sprouts of this plant in spring in order to make themselves strong and healthy during the ensuing year.

3. Hilis hàtki, "white medicine." This is ginseng and it was a very highly esteemed remedy. Caley Proctor said that when one suffered from shortness of breath the roots of this plant were cut up and put into boiling water and the infusion drunk. It was not used externally. Jackson Lewis also mentioned its use in cases of shortness of breath, and he added croup in children and a very low general condition. It constituted one of the elements in many compound remedies and generally relieved the patient. When a person was sick with fever and could not sweat new ginseng was boiled with ginger, then both were mixed with alcohol and a little given to the patient, when sweat would break out all over him. It was also used, according to both Caley Proctor and Jackson Lewis, to stop the flow of blood from a cut. The latter by its means cured a woman who had been shot in the head. Before applying the medicine in such cases the wound was cleaned out by the use of the long wing feather of a buzzard. At that time no one must be near, especially no woman, and above all a woman at the time of her monthly period. Elsewhere I have mentioned its employment to keep away ghosts, and Adair says "the Indians use it on religious occasions." [40]

Caley Proctor gave me the following formula used over this medicine in cases of shortness of breath:

> nokī' saladī' nokī' łe'slai salatī'
> nokī' łesfánk salatī' kaka' kaka'

It is not known whether the words have any meaning. When this medicine is used to stop the flow of blood from cuts the following meaningless formula is hummed:

> katadàs howē' kati lanidī'
> apàtánalanidī' saii

---

[37] Adair, Hist. Am. Inds., p. 103.
[38] Swan in Schoolcraft, Ind. Tribes, vol. v, p. 268.
[39] Adair, op. cit., pp. 102–103.
[40] Ibid., p. 362. It was employed, for instance, during the busk at Kasihta (see p. 578).

SWANTON]   CREEK RELIGION AND MEDICINE   **657**

4. Notosa. This is the angelica, the roots of which were used in various physical ailments. Bartram calls it "the angelica lucida or nondo," and says "it is in high estimation with the Indians as well as with the white inhabitants, and sells at a great price to the Southern Indians of Florida, who dwell near the sea coast where this never grows spontaneously."[41] In another place he remarks that "its friendly carminitive qualities are well known for relieving all the disorders of the stomach, a dry belly-ache and disorders of the intestines, colic, hysterics, etc. The patient chews the root and swallows the juice, or smokes it when dry with tobacco. Even the smell of the root is of good effect. The Lower Creeks (Semmole), in whose country it does not grow, will gladly give two or three buckskins for a single root of it."[42] According to Jackson Lewis it was given to children as a vermifuge and to adults to alleviate pains in the back.

5. Wilāna. This is the wormseed (*Chenopodium ambrosioides*). It was used to purify the busk ground and in the final cleansing of the fasters at that time. According to Caley Proctor it was a kind of family medicine, apparently a sort of spring tonic, and was also used in cases of fever. Jackson Lewis said it was employed in a great many ailments.

6. Atcina, cedar. According to Caley Proctor cedar was used as a spring tonic, to thin the blood. The Alabama in Texas bandaged it, after it had been boiled, over a place where there were rheumatic pains. According to Jackson Lewis the sprigs and leaves were applied warm to places where pains and aches were felt. It was not taken internally.

7. Kȧpapȧska, spicewood (*Benzoin aestivale*). When pains and aches were experienced an infusion was made of the branches and taken internally or the body steamed in the liquid in order to produce a perspiration. It was also taken in conjunction with miko hoyanīdja to produce vomiting, "which after some time purifies the blood greatly." Sometimes it was used as we use tea.

8. Kofûtcka låko, horsemint (a species of *Monarda*). The entire plant was used in an infusion in order to bring on a perspiration. When one was delirious he could be cured by the use of horsemint and everlasting boiled together and administered internally. According to Caley Proctor it was boiled with miko hoyanīdja to cure dropsy and swellings in the legs. The patient drank it hot and also bathed in it. The Alabama called it tcinok tiłaile, and it was used after a person had died, to ward off the rheumatism which was likely to ensue and also to cure all kinds of rheumatism. It was mixed with cold water, conjured by the doctor, and then each member of the household washed his body in it up to the ears, besides drinking some. It was used on the morning or evening after the death and was for protection against the ghost of the dead, which otherwise might afflict one with deafness.

---
[41] Bartram, Travels, p. 325.
[42] Trans. Am. Ethnol. Soc., vol. III, p. 47.

9. Kadohwa, honey locust. This is used not to cure disease but to ward it off. The sprigs, thorns, and some of the branches are chopped up quite fine and boiled in water. After the infusion has been thoroughly boiled the members of the family bathe in it to ward off contagions such as smallpox and measles. It should be employed for four successive days.

10. Ala (Alabama ayona), buckeye (*Aesculus*). This is a very strong medicine and but little can be taken at a time. The roots are employed in cases of pulmonary consumption. It is also used to stupefy fishes.

11. Aloniski or holoniski, the devil's shoestring (*Cracca virginiana*). Jackson Lewis said that this was used in the same way as the buckeye and for the same purpose. Caley Proctor said that eight roots were pounded up, mixed with water, and the resultant infusion drunk cold in cases of bladder trouble. Together with yelungadjādi it was used in cases of loss of manhood, being prepared in the same manner. Like the preceding, it was employed to stupefy fish.

12. Adokłá lásti, "black weed" (*Baptisia*), has a papilionaceous flower, yellow in color, and grows in clumps to a height of 2½ to 3 feet. The roots of this plant were boiled in water and administered to children who seemed drowsy and lifeless and on the point of coming down with some sickness. They were bathed in it and a little was given to them to drink.

13. Tcato hiliswa, "rock medicine," grows in clumps and has a beautiful blue flower which appears early in spring. The roots are hard to get out and are as bitter as quinine. It was not used like the other medicines but apparently only when the old medicine men were making the novices fast.

14. Yanasa hiliswa, "bison medicine." It was formerly customary to put some medicine made from the roots of this on the tongue of a newborn child to make him strong, robust, and daring. Some of it grows in the old Choctaw country.

15. Tcito yektca hiliswa, "medicine of the strong snake" (sarsaparilla). The roots were used when there was difficulty in urinating and blood was passed and there was pain about the lower part of the abdomen and in the back. Eakins says they resorted to it in cases of pleurisy.[43] The Choctaw and Chickasaw also use it, but they have a different name for the plant.

16. Sokha hiliswa, "hog medicine," boneset (apparently). When women complained of aches and pains in the hips they were steamed in a medicine made by boiling this. The Choctaw and Chickasaw called it cilup tiłeli, which means "something to scare away the spirits." A decoction was made from the roots and when persons had epilepsy they were steamed in it.

---

[43] Schoolcraft, Ind. Tribes, vol. I, p. 274.

17. Tuhiligu, mistletoe (*Phoradendron flavescens*). The leaves and branches were used as one of the ingredients in medicines for lung trouble, consumption, etc.

18. Akhātka, "white down in" (the bottom), the sycamore (*Platanus occidentalis*). Chips from the tree and bark were used to make a medicine taken internally in cases of pulmonary tuberculosis. The following three medicines were used for the same purpose:

19. Aktcelalāskă the white birch (*Betula*) of Oklahoma.

20. Tculi niha, (yellow) "pine rosin."

21. Hikŭlwă, the black gum (*Nyssa*). The bark and chips of the wood were boiled and the decoction taken internally, or else the patient was bathed in it.

22. Tawa tcāti, "red sumac." This is the smooth sumac (*Rhus glabra*). The roots were boiled and the infusion taken internally in cases of dysentery. It was the leaves of this variety which they formerly mixed with their smoking tobacco, and Pope says "this preparation of *Sumach* and *Tobacco*, the *Indians* constantly smoke, and consider as a sovereign Remedy in all cephalic and pectoral Complaints." [44]

23. Tawa lăsti, "black sumac" (*Rhus copallina*). The roots were used like those of the preceding.

24. Ahwāna, willow (Alabama, ito loica). The roots were boiled in water and the infusion kept in the house in the summertime so that the family might bathe in it and drink it and thereby ward off fevers.

The Texas Alabama used this to cure fevers. The roots were put into cold water, and the doctor came every morning for four mornings and blew into the infusion, after which the patient drank of it and bathed in it all over.

25. Kī, mulberry (*Morus rubra*) (Alabama, bihala). The roots were used as an emetic. The Texas Alabama boiled and drank an infusion of these roots four or five times a day in cases of weakness accompanied by the passage of very yellow urine.

26. Tcoskă, post oak (*Quercus stellata*). The bark is used to make a drink which Jackson Lewis used in cases of dysentery. Other physicians employed it in various other ways, but he did not know how.

27. Păkānaho, the wild plum (*Prunus*). The roots were boiled in water, and the infusion was taken internally in cases of dysentery.

28. Itco impăkānă, "deer's apple," a kind of wild crabapple (*Malus*). Jackson Lewis believed he had cured numerous persons of hydrophobia by taking the patient as soon as possible after he had been bitten, boiling some of this until a strong decoction had been made, and having the patient drink frequently of it, besides bathing him in the liquid and steaming the wound with it.

[44] Pope Tour, p. 63.

29. Tàfōso, elm (*Ulmus*). Jackson Lewis knew that this was used in cases of toothache and he thought that the branches were taken, but there was a secret about its use which the doctors who knew about it did not divulge and he was not acquainted with it.

30. Pàłko łàko, "big grape," the "summer grape." The use of this in snake bite has been mentioned already.[45] It was also employed in cases of tonsilitis, when the tendrils were steeped in hot water and cloths put into this and bound about the throat. With it must be little parings of ginseng.

31. Hayopalīdjà łàko, the wild rose. The roots were boiled and administered internally to women when they were irregular in their periods.

32. Hayopalīdjà tcutci, a dwarf variety of wild rose. The roots of this were used with sumac in cases of dysentery. Either this or the preceding was employed by the Natchez in similar cases. My informant could not recall the Natchez name, but it is named in Cherokee tsistuunigist uhsti, "little rabbit food."

33. Tałdakà, cottonwood (*Populus*). When an arm or leg had been broken cottonwood bark was boiled and the resulting liquid poured over the fractured part. Splints were made from the inner bark of this tree and it is asserted that the bone would then knit very soon. It was also used when ankles or other joints were sprained. If this tree is identical with the ito tàsikaya, or "warrior tree," it was also used in cases of dropsy, when the patient was bathed in an infusion made by boiling the roots.

34. Adàphà, dogwood (*Cornus*). Jackson Lewis had seen this used but had never employed it himself and had forgotten the nature of its supposed virtues. The Texas Alabama, however, boiled the inner bark of the dogwood and used it in cases of flux.

35. Imbàkbàki tcati, "red blossoms," a plant growing in clumps in Oklahoma, with strong, rough, tuberous roots which are used as medicine in cases of pneumonia and to bring on perspiration and secure a reaction in what is called "winter fever." The bunches of this plant sometimes have red flowers and sometimes yellow ones.

36. Tinetki hiliswa, "thunder medicine," has very bitter roots and is used in fevers.

37. Itco imaha, "deer's potato," a *Lacinaria*, was used to cure the deer disease—i. e., rheumatism. The roots were pounded up and boiled, and the infusion rubbed on the affected parts. Some was also drunk. According to Jackson Lewis pàsa was used in connection with it and a little sprig of cedar was also put in. Caley Proctor did not mention these accessories.

38. Hitci omà, "like tobacco," mullen (*Verbascum thapsus*). The roots were boiled and used internally for coughs, but there must be added to them the roots of a plant growing in wet places called

---

45 See p. 645.

"button willow" in English and by the Creeks sáksa imito, "crawfish wood." This last reaches a height of 5 or 6 feet. The identification of this is somewhat doubtful as I showed a piece of mullen to Caley Proctor and he called it waga inhidji and said it was used for shooting pains in the chest and joints. The leaves were boiled and the patient bathed in the infusion while it was still hot.

39. Tcokiliba, the elderberry .(*Sambucus canadensis*). The tender roots of this plant were pounded up, stirred into hot water, and bound on the breast of a woman suffering from a swollen breast. If the roots can not be gotten, the skin scraped off of the stalk may be employed.

40. Katco łáko, "big briar," the greenbriar (*Smilax*). The roots of this plant, which are exceedingly hard, are pounded up, boiled, and the liquid poured over ulcers, particularly ulcers on the legs.

41. Ahálobaktsi, or Halobáktci, *Gnaphalium obtusifolium*, was used, according to Jackson Lewis, in cases of mumps. A great many leaves were collected, even in winter when they are dried up, a strong infusion was made by boiling them in water, cloths were dipped in this, a little lard added, and the whole tied around the throat. According to Caley Proctor this was put with several other medicines, among which he mentioned atcīna, miko hoyanīdja, pāsa, wīlana, and kofutcka łáko, to add a perfume. They were boiled by themselves, and the infusion drunk when one was unable to keep anything upon the stomach. The patient also bathed in the liquid. To cure bad colds the tops were boiled, the odor inhaled, and the infusion drunk. The faces and heads of old people were bathed in it and some drunk when they could not rest well and woke up with a start as soon as they had fallen asleep.

42. Iswiani tcaitcga, "a purgative" (the only name known) (*Euphorbia*?). This is a small weed with small smooth leaves, and bears a bunch of flowers at the top. When broken it exudes a little milk. The roots are taken in an infusion to bring on an action of the bowels and it is a very violent remedy.

43. Wīso, sassafras (*Sassafras variifolium*). This was used as a medicine but I have no information as to how it was employed.

44. Puya fiktca hiliswa, "spirit medicine," is a weed a foot high which produces a little yellow fruit just where the leaf comes away from the stalk. This is said to be very fine for rheumatism and it is declared that it will cure gonorrhea. A bundle of roots is taken sufficiently large to fill the palm in the space inclosed by the thumb and second finger when the tips are brought together.

45. Bittersweet (*Celastrus scandens*). Jackson Lewis knew no native name for this plant. It is good for women with urinary troubles or having pains about the small of the back. The person taking this medicine must not eat butter, milk, or bacon.

46. Afála oma, "like the ivy," the woodbine (*Parthenocissus*). The root of this is good medicine in cases of gonorrhea. Its use was learned from the Comanche.

47. Stilást iga ("black man's medicine"), a plant with a yellow flower popularly known as "nigger head." The roots were boiled and used in cases of consumption.

48. Pisi hiliswa, "woman's-breast medicine," a plant the roots of which were mashed, mixed with warm water, and applied externally by women suffering from swollen breasts.

49. Ifulo hiliswa, "screech owl medicine," is found far out in the woods, growing in small bunches. An entire bunch was boiled so that the infusion might be as strong as possible. The water then turns red and is good for persons with watery eyes or other chronic eye troubles.

50. Kīstowa, known popularly to the whites as "red root," a woody shrub with leaves along the stem and hard, woody, red roots. The roots are cut into long strips and put into a bottle with cold water. Afterwards the infusion is employed when blood is spit from the lungs.

51. Hitci pákpági ("tobacco bloom"), native tobacco, some species of lobelia(?). This is said to grow to a height of about 10 inches, but otherwise to resemble the common tobacco exactly and to have the same kind of flower. Jackson Lewis said that he knew that the Creeks, Yuchi, and Shawnee had this but was not aware of its existence among any other Indians. It is of rare occurrence and very highly valued. Traditionally this plant was with the Creeks from the very beginning, and it is supposed to be older than the smoking tobacco. Nevertheless Tuggle seems to have preserved a myth recounting its origin.[45a] It derives its name from the fact that the flowers were the part used in medicine, four of them being generally placed in the pot. It was used in all kinds of cases, sometimes when a person was sick to the point of delirium, and it was used to ward off ghosts. Incidental references to this medicine have been made in other places.

The following medicines were described to me by Caley Proctor:

52. Awanhi hiliswa. This plant grows to a height of about 3 feet and bears a yellow flower. It is not used externally, but the roots are boiled and the infusion drunk to cure an enlarged spleen.

53. Yelungádjádi hiliswa, a species of *Stillingia*, is a plant about a foot and a half tall and has a bushy top with no blossom, or probably an inconspicuous one. The roots were mashed and boiled and a woman who had just given birth to a child drank the liquid and was bathed in it. A woman suffering from irregular periods bathed in this, prepared with the addition of devil's shoestring.

45a See p. 509.

54. Fatdjådjī has a bunchy top, small yellow flowers, and short, very white roots. These last were boiled in water and the mixture drunk hot in cases of flux. When a small baby is very weak it is made to drink some of this and it is bathed in it.

55. Totkop låko, a species of *Impatiens*, is boiled with kofûtcka låko and spicewood and the mixture drunk hot in cases of dropsy. The patient also bathes in it.

56. Nuti hiliswa, "tooth medicine," yarrow (*Achillea millefolium*), was used, as its name implies, to cure any sort of toothache.

For some diseases objects shaped like the old atasa or war club were put into medicines. A white man long acquainted with the Indians said that one kind of treatment was to pour great quantities of cold water over the patient. Liver complaint is called in Creek wī'ak wiligi.

ALABAMA MEDICINES

57. Nåtikåca litcī, "cooler of the teeth," *Zanthoxylum americanum* Mill., popularly known as "prickly ash." The inside bark was beaten up and some of it was inserted into the cavity in an aching tooth, while more was placed around it and the whole wrapped up in a cloth. If a person itched all over, some was boiled in a pot and rubbed over him. When a man was out hunting and his dog did not follow the trail well he would sometimes put some of this bark into cold water and rub the dog's nose with it to improve his scent.

58. Håk-himbålka, "wild goose's berries," *Callicarpa americana*, popularly called the French mulberry. The roots and limbs were put into a pot together, boiled, and then poured into a big pan. This was then placed beside a person suffering from malarial fever ("sick one day and well the next") in a sweat house made like that of the Creeks. After he had perspired all over he came out and was bathed in water. The treatment was repeated until the patient was cured. Sometimes the pan was placed beneath the chair of a person having rheumatism and blankets were then fastened about him. This was also to induce perspiration and it was repeated four times if necessary. Slow fever was treated in the same manner but my informant assured me that it was unsuccessful in such cases, as he himself had tried it.

59. Comalī, a species of *Meibomia*, the popular name of which is "tick trefoil." A bad state of the lungs or sometimes a bad cold was cured by drinking a tea made of this before breakfast and then vomiting it up.

60. Ahisi låksa, "bitter or strong medicine," *Gnaphalium obtusifolium* L., popularly known as "rabbit tobacco."[46] Låksa indicates a taste between bitter and sour. This was often used mixed with other medicines, but my informant did not know what. It was used, furthermore, when a man was nervous, woke up frequently, and

---

[46] There is doubt of this, as the same name is given to an *Antennaria*, popularly known as "pussy toes."

wanted to run away. It was then boiled in water along with cedar and the face of the patient washed in it until he got well. This sickness was thought to be brought on by ghosts and the medicine was intended to drive them off. Another way to effect the same end was by burning this plant and cedar together.

61. Hátācipa, or Háthācipá, a species of *Solidago*, popularly known as "goldenrod," A tea was made out of the roots and drunk to cure a bad cold. Sometimes the root, which is bitter, was put into the cavity in a tooth to stop the ache.

62. Yenasa imilpa, "buffalo eat it," *Ceanothus americanus* L., the popular name of which is "New Jersey tea." The roots were boiled in water for two or three hours, the whole allowed to cool, and then it was used to bathe the feet or legs of one who had been injured in those members. This was done three times a day for one week, two weeks, or even for a month—i. e., until the injury was healed.

63. Wásáko'tcī, a species of *Vaccinium*, the blueberry. It was used as a remedy for many different ailments but my informant did not know what these were.

64. Nita imilpa, "bears eat it," has black berries. It was used for the same purposes as the Nátikāca litcī and in the same way. A poultice was made from it and applied in cases of pneumonia.

65. Ito hici' kocōma, "fragrant leaves," the sweet bay (*Myrica*). This was put into a big pot along with another medicine, perhaps cedar, and boiled. It was then administered to a person after a burial had taken place in order to secure him from disease. He did not retain it in his stomach, but went outside and vomited it up, after which he could eat.

66. Omágāga, "open eyes," *Ascyrum multicaule*, popular name "St. Peter's-wort." When one had a bad case of dysentery these plants were put into a pot entire and boiled for a long time, and the infusion taken cold four or five times a day. In two or three days the patient would get better. It derives its name from the fact that a tea was also made from it with which to wash out the eyes.

67. Hācā'lápo. The twirling stick used in producing fire in ancient times was made from this. A tea was made from the stalk and leaves of it, and given internally and externally to a person suffering from a disease locally known as "the itch," which seems to be prickly heat, shingles, or something of the kind.

68. Tcūyi, the pine. The inside bark of pine saplings was boiled in water and drunk to cure flux.

69. Ahisi home, "bitter medicine." The roots and the inside bark of the stalk were beaten up and put into water. After soaking thoroughly the medicine was tied up in a clean cloth and placed over any part of the body where a pain was felt, which it relieved, although it raised a blister. It was also put against the cheek outside of an aching tooth in order to destroy the pain—sometimes into the cavity of the tooth itself.

70. Itichǎlōkpa, the holly (*Ilex*). The inside bark was scraped off
and boiled for a long time, perhaps four hours, in water, after which it
was applied to sore eyes as a wash. It was administered three or
four times a day.

71. Łatco, red oak. The bark was boiled, and in the morning
before food had been taken the infusion was drunk and then vomited
out by a person afflicted with lung trouble. It was sometimes used to
wash bad smelling sores that had broken out on the feet or the head.
When children old enough to walk were too weak to do so, red oak
bark, tree moss, omágāga, and oyimpák'o (tall bushes which grow
near rocks) were mashed up together and boiled in a pot and the
whole used as a wash. Sometimes a doctor was employed in connection with this; sometimes not. Boiled red-oak bark was also
resorted to in cases of sore throat.

72. Tǎkǎctaya, or Tǎkǎstǎyǎ, *Cercis canadensis* L., popularly
known as the "redbud" or "Judas tree." The roots and inside bark
were put into a small bucket with water where they were sometimes
conjured by the doctor and sometimes not. The mixture was then
drunk from four to six times a day to cure a kind of "congestion"
which causes one to become hot all over and is soon fatal if not
checked.

73. Ahisi hǎtka, "white medicine," perhaps ginseng. The roots
were broken off and the milk that comes from them rubbed on sores.

74. Bǎkca, bark of the slippery elm (*Ulmus fulva*). When a woman
was in labor and the delivery was delayed this was sometimes administered to her after it had been boiled in water along with gunpowder.
The reasons assigned involve sympathetic magic.

75. Iłopotle, "acting on or moving [the bowels]," *Sebastiana
ligustrina* (Michx.) Muell. The roots of this were chewed to produce
a movement of the bowels.

76. Dropsy was treated as follows: A limb was taken from the
east side of each of four trees. These were put into a pot of water
and boiled and the patient given a sweat bath. When he perspired
profusely all over, he was washed in the same medicine and dressed
in clean clothes. The same thing was repeated three times every
day until he got well. Every morning, while this was going on, the
doctor came and blew into the medicine. It was done for four
successive days and if the treatment was ineffective it was repeated.

77. White-flour corn. To treat slow fever they pounded up four
kernels of flour corn, mixed them with water, and poured the whole
through a sieve held over the patient's head until all was gone. Next
day the doctor did the same thing over again, calling upon the North,
West, South, and East, blowing into the medicine and pouring it
over the patient. Afterwards the patient's body was rubbed in
order to bleach it, and that is why the white flour corn was used.

In this way the soul of the sick man which was supposed to have gone up to the sky was recalled to its body.

78. Itco intcástuge, "deer's peas," *Erythrina herbacea*. The roots were pounded up, put into water, and the infusion drunk cold by a woman who had pains in the bowels.

79. Kátsgimilpa, "catfish eat it," or "catfish food." This is the famous "black drink" or "cassine" (*Ilex vomitoria*) referred to by all early writers on the southern Indians. The Creeks commonly called it ási, meaning simply "leaves," but sawátcka is said by some to have been the true name.[46a] However, there appears to be some difference of opinion about this. I did not learn of any strictly medicinal purpose to which it was put by either the Alabama or the Creeks, though it was daily employed by the old people in early days to clear out the system and produce ceremonial purity. That it was supposed to possess more specific curative properties is shown by the following quotation from Adair:

"The Yopon, or Cusseena, is very plenty, as far as the salt air reaches over the low lands. It is well tasted, and very agreeable to those who accustom themselves to use it; instead of having any noxious quality, according to what many have experienced of the East-India insipid and costly tea, it is friendly to the human system, enters into a contest with the peccant humours, and expels them through the various channels of nature: it perfectly cures a tremor in the nerves." [47]

A toothache medicine was known to an old woman, now dead, living among the Alabama in Texas but belonging herself to the Biloxi or Pascagoula tribe. It is said to be only a few inches tall and to have a red blossom. Mrs. James McKee, wife of the farmer with whom I boarded while in Texas, told me that "old Sally," as this woman was called, had cured a toothache for her almost instantly by putting some of the root of this plant into the cavity. The first application was accompanied by intense pain which soon disappeared and never returned. Apparently the nerve had been killed. Afterwards she asked the old woman repeatedly to show her the plant but the latter refused to do so lest it should lose its efficacy.

NATCHEZ MEDICINES

The following medicines were enumerated to me by one of the few surviving Natchez Indians. As the latter are living among the Cherokee it is probable that they are as much Cherokee as Natchez, and indeed for some of them I could obtain only the Cherokee names. Unless otherwise stated, the native name is in Natchez.

80. Cherokee name kowaya yūst', "syphilis medicine," a species of *Ascyrum* popularly known as St. Andrew's cross. A tea was made from it and given to children unable to pass urine.

[46a] Possibly sawátcka is from ási, "leaves," and awotaitcita, "to make vomit," or sawotka, "emetic."
[47] Adair, Hist. Am. Inds., p. 361.

81. Paxpa'ugubic, *Triosteum perfoliatum*, popularly know.1 as horse gentian and locally as pleurisy root. While this was a medicine plant, my informant did not know how it was employed.

82. This is a species of *Asclepias* popularly known as milkweed. My informant did not know of a native name for it either in Natchez or Cherokee. The root was cut into several small pieces, a tea made from them, and three swallows taken three times a day for four days to cure kidney trouble and Bright's disease. Meantime the patient must take nothing that contained salt.[47a]

83. Cherokee name antnáx iyūsti, "strawberry like," *Potentilla canadensis*, popularly called cinquefoil. This was given to one who had been bewitched.

84. We-bulu, *Smilax bona-nox*, popularly called cat briar. This stays green all winter, and so it is wet and rubbed on the face to make one young.

85. Tsoliyux, *Aristolochia serpentaria*. The whole plant is put into water and boiled, after which the infusion is taken internally while still warm to cure fevers.

86. Awel dáxdau[n], "dangerous plant," *Leptotaenia nuttallii*. If this plant is eaten in winter it is said that it will prove fatal because at that season the snakes put poison into it, but in summer it is used as a medicine, though my informant did not know for what diseases.

87. Cherokee name Táloni yuxsti, perhaps from a town in the old country known as Tálonigi [Dahlonega], (*Rhus trilobata*). The roots are gathered and kept all winter, and if a poultice is made from them and put over a boil it is certain to kill it.

88. Ooc bobátsihīc, "owl shoe," *Camassia esculenta*, popularly called quamash. It was used as a medicine but my informant could not say for what.

89. A species of *Porteranthus*, the Natchez and Cherokee names of which my informant could not give, nor did he himself know for what it was used, although he remembered having seen the old women hunting for it when he was a boy. He thought it might have been used by women during their monthly periods.

90. Cherokee name Ihiya yūst', "like cane," a species of *Panicum*, popularly called panic grass. An infusion was drunk warm to cure fevers which return every other day—i. e., malaria—and it was drunk hot for steady fevers.

91. Tsu ha'yax, *Rhamnus caroliniana*. Four blocks of wood were taken from this tree and a tea made out of them which was drunk for jaundice.

92. Cherokee name Gáhûnski, a species of *Pentstemon*. The *Collinsia violacea* is considered to be a smaller species of the same thing. A tea was made from the roots and administered to cure whooping cough, consumption, coughs, and colds.

[47a] This is probably identical with No. 93, though it may be a different species.

93. A species of *Asclepias* popularly called "milkweed." No native name could be remembered. This was used in cases of syphilis.[47b]

94. Căxwăł. This is perhaps *Vernonia*, popularly known as ironweed. A tea was made out of the whole plant and drunk in cases of dysentery.

95. Wenădu ici, "cat's tail." This is still unidentified. A tea was made of the whole plant and was used like the preceding in cases of dysentery.

96. Agwenăhimbok, a species of *Antennaria*, popularly known as pussy toes (see p. 664). A tea was made from the tops and roots together and drunk warm to cure coughs and colds.

97. Awel abociił, *Northoscordum bivalve*, a relative of the wild onions. This was probably used as a medicine also, but my informant did not say for what.

98. Cedar (mōgăt) was used for pains in the shoulders, breast and back, for mumps, and swellings in the legs.

99. A root called by my informants the "pleurisy or butterfly root" is declared to have been as good a remedy as could be found for pneumonia or winter fever. The roots were boiled and the infusion taken a teacupful at a time. If one sick with a hot dry fever drank this and wrapped himself up well in bed he would soon perspire freely.

100. The "button snake-root" (āwelwaih; Creek, pāsa) is a great remedy for nosebleed. If the stem and leaves were chewed it would stop the flow of blood. A tea made of the parched plants was good for flux. After imbibing it the patient would fast until sundown and then make himself vomit. In olden days it is said to have been used instead of salt.

101. The entire plant of the long winter fern (tsōgōbīc, "bear paw;" Cherokee, "bear bed") was used as a remedy for scurvy.

102. The red willow (ōm bāgup, "red medicine"; Creek, miko hoyanīdja) was used for fevers.

103. The wormseed (ōm tsucgop, "strong-smelling medicine"; Creek, wīlānă) was given to people with fever or to children having worms.

104. "The devil's shoestring" (ănūh tsānuh) was thought to be good for coughs. As among the Creeks, it was also used in poisoning fish.

105. A plant growing to a height of 2 or 3 feet on the uplands and 5 in the bottoms, with hollow stems reaching the size of a lead pencil, and a yellowish flower, is esteemed good for the liver (or spleen) and for pains in the side.

Songs with appropriate words must be employed in administering all of the above medicines.

[47b] Probably identical with No. 82, though possibly a different species.

When a man became sick at the stomach and vomited it was believed that a dead person had been eating out of the same dish with him.

Water from certain springs was also used as a remedy.   There is a prairie in the Cherokee Nation formerly known as Medicine Spring Prairie (Gun ōm gunáts) but now called Greenleaf Prairie (Tsu otol hāyáp).   The medicine spring from which it was originally named is 4 miles east of Braggs and the water is good for rheumatism, fevers, backache, headache, pains in the breast or stomach, weak or sore eyes, and has especial value for children.   The water makes one belch a great deal, and "when you first drink it you do not like it but after a time you get used to it and think it the finest water in the world."

In the mountains 5 or 6 miles farther east is another spring with the very same kind of water, and a third 2 to 3 miles above Gore, on the bank of the Illinois River.   A long time ago the Indians used to throw things into these.

To these may be added some mention of medicines by early writers.   Adair speaks of an aquatic plant, probably a species of yellow flowered water lily (*Nymphaea*), the seeds of which were used as food.   After noting this fact he continues: "It is a sort of marsh-mallows, and reckoned a speedy cure for burning maladies, either outward or inward—for the former, by an outward application of the leaf; and for the latter, by a decoction of it drank plentifully."   He adds that the Choctaw called one of their head towns by its name.[48]

Swan says: "The cassia fistularius, or pod of the wild locust, which grows here in abundance, furnishes them late in autumn with a kind of sweetmeats, which they gather and bring home wherever they can find it; and it is esteemed a good antidote in the complaints of their children."[49]   It is quite certain that this is in reality the honey locust (*Gleditsia triacanthos*).

After mentioning whooping cough and worms as diseases from which Creek children frequently suffered Bartram says: "But (besides their well-known remedy, *Spigelia anthelmintica*), to prevent the troublesome and fatal effects of this disease, they use a strong *lixivium* prepared from ashes of bean-stalks and other vegetables, in all their food prepared from corn (*zea*), which otherwise, they say, breeds worms in their stomachs."[50]

Below we read: "The vegetables which I discovered to be used as remedies, were generally very powerful cathartics.   Of this class are several species of the *Iris*, viz, *Ir. versicolor*, *Ir. verna*.   And for the same purpose they have a high estimation of a species of either *Croton* or *Styllingia*, I am in doubt which."   He adds that this last

[48] Adair, Hist. Am. Inds., p. 410.   I have been unable to identify the name of the town.

[49] Schoolcraft, Ind. Tribes, vol. v, p. 270.

[50] Bartram, Trans. Am. Eth. Soc., vol. III, p. 43.

had been used very successfully by a white physician in North Carolina "in curing the *yaws.*" [51]

Still farther on he says: "Several species of *Smilax,* the woody vines of *Bignonia crucigera,* some of the *bays* (*laurus*), are of great account with the Indians as remedies . . .

"The caustic and detergent properties of the white nettle (roots) of Carolina and Florida (*Jatropha urens*), used for cleansing old ulcers and consuming proud-flesh, and likewise the dissolvent and diuretant powers of the root of the convolvulus panduratus [*Ipomoea pandurata*], so much esteemed as a remedy in nephritic complaints, were discovered by the Indians to the inhabitants of Carolina." [52]

One or two other items may be added from notes taken by the Agent Eakins from an Alabama Indian:

"The big prairie-weed is used as an emetic, taken as a tea. For cathartics they have a number of roots and weeds, prepared as a tea . . . They have two modes of treating eruptions of the skin: First, the external application of a decoction of herbs; and, Secondly, by steaming with the same decoction. The cause of their known and general failure to treat small-pox, or varioloid, is, First, their limited knowledge of the nature of the disease; and, Secondly, their belief that it is contagious prevents their administering for its cure. In no cases, whatever, do men assist in parturition. After parturition, they use a simple root or weed. For paralysis, their treatment is not, in all cases, successful, which is generally by roots or herbs. They use the vapor bath efficaciously." [53]

SUPPLEMENTARY NOTE

Through the kindness of Mr. David I. Bushnell, Jr., I am able to add the following notes regarding a Creek busk witnessed by the artist J. M. Stanley and Mr. Sumner Dickerman in the summer of 1843, the year after the busk described by General Hitchcock. They were contained in a letter written at "Bayou Menard, Cherokee Nation, August 4, 1843," by Mr. Dickerman and printed in a newspaper, and give little more than an account—a very good one nevertheless—of the women's dance. The town was probably Tukabahchee, but this is uncertain. Mr. Dickerman, as well as his companion, seems to have had some artistic ability, since the services of both gentlemen were utilized by the Indians in painting a banner for the occasion. "On one side was painted the American Eagle, with the motto, 'E Pluribus Unum,' and the thirteen stars; on the other the crossed pipes, hatchet, and clasped hands, with the motto of 'Peace and Friendship.'" After Mr. Dickerman had run this up on a pole about 21 feet high, at one corner of the square, the Indians took it down and inverted it so that the eagle might be seen from the inside of the square as the wind was then blowing.

Mr. Dickerman describes the ceremonial ground as measuring "about 35 feet square," and says, "on each side is a small house with open front, facing the interior, and an entrance from each end of the house. Seats were arranged in

---

[51] Bartram, Trans. Am. Eth. Soc., p. 44.

[52] Ibid., pp. 44–47.

[53] Schoolcraft, Ind. Tribes, vol. I, p. 274.

each house made of matting of cane wove together with bark. In the centre of the square they have a fire, which is not suffered to go out during the year. At the time of the *Busk* every family in the town is obliged to put out their fire at home and go to the Busking ground and encamp." He was, as we know, misinformed regarding the fire, which was kept up only during the ceremonial period. He now proceeds to describe the doings of the first day as follows:

"The *Busk* is a religious ceremony, to return thanks to the Great Spirit for their abundant crops of Corn, and might be called their sacrament, as it is observed with the utmost strictness and self-denial. The first day of the ceremony was commenced by the women dancing. They gave us the highest seat in the synagogue, where we could see every thing that was going on. The little King, or Chief of the town, with three others, took their seats upon the cane mats at one corner of the square, and in a few moments after they were seated, four gourds were brought to them on a server made of cane, which was painted white with a kind of clay, and contained small round seeds. Each man took one and they then commenced singing and keeping time with the gourds, the women at the same time coming into the square in Indian file, marched up in front and faced the singers. After they had come in to the number of one hundred and fifty, the singing ceased, and the speaker gave them a 'talk,' the substance of which, I am sorry to say I am unable to give you, as we had no interpreter by us at that time. At the conclusion of the speech the singing again commenced, and the four old women who led the dance, each holding a stick about a foot long, painted red and ornamented with Eagle's feathers, commenced beating time. The King gave a signal by the shake of the gourd, and they all immediately faced about and commenced beating time with their feet. About fifty of them wore terrapin shells upon their legs, which are made in the following manner: They boil the terrapin, extract all the meat, and then fill it with small pebble stones. Ten or twelve of these are fastened in a semicircular form upon a piece of Buffalo skin, and tied upon the leg just above the knee. They generally wear one on each leg, and in dancing they all keep perfect time, and it is impossible to conceive what a rattling noise they make. Another double shake of the gourd, and they all commenced dancing around the fire in the centre of the square. In this way they continued dancing incessantly for two hours, the sun shining full upon them, and the thermometer ranging from 90 to 100 in the shade. Their dresses defy description. Out of the whole number I could not designate two of the same figure. They were principally of calico and cotton of their own manufacture. They were made in a style peculiar to the Creeks and Seminoles. The border is made to hang loose, and detached from the skirt. The skirt is tied around the waist, and is worked to the depth of 12 or 15 inches from the bottom with different colors, in various devices. On these occasions they always put on all and the best they have. I saw one woman near our camp put on five dresses. They wore a great many ornaments, such as beads, ear-rings, hair-combs, etc. I saw one woman with ten pair of silver ear-rings in her ears, four pounds of large blue and white beads around her neck, silver armbands upon her arms, and about ten yards of different colored ribbons flowing from the top of her head. While the women were dancing the men were all seated in the houses forming the square, feasting upon boiled meat, potatoes, honey and water-mellons. They asked us if we had eaten any green corn this season; we replied that we had. They then told us if we had not eaten corn we could have eaten with them, but if we had eaten of it we could not, for it would spoil their physic, and offend the Great Spirit. Thus passed the first day of the Busk. . . ."

Dickerman promises to continue his description of the ceremony in later letters but unfortunately they are not available to me.

BIBLIOGRAPHY

ADAIR, JAMES. The history of the American Indians. London, 1775.
BARTRAM, WM. Observations on the Creek and Cherokee Indians. 1789. With prefatory and supplementary notes by E. G. Squier. Trans. Amer. Ethn. Soc., vol. III, pt. 1, New York, 1853.

——— Travels through North and South Carolina, Georgia, East and West Florida, the Cherokee country, the extensive territories of the Muscogulges or Creek Confederacy, and the country of the Chactaws. London, 1792.
BOSOMWORTH, THOMAS. Journal of 1752. (Ms. in South Carolina archives; copy in archives of Bur. Amer. Ethn.)
BOSSU, M. Nouveaux Voyages aux Indes Occidentales. Vols. I–II. Paris, 1768.
CLAIBORNE, J. F. H. Mississippi as a Province, Territory, and State. Vol. I [only volume printed]. Jackson, 1880.
DU PRATZ. See Le Page du Pratz.
GATSCHET, ALBERT S. A migration legend of the Creek Indians. Vol. I, Phila., 1884 [Brinton's Library of Aboriginal American Literature, No. 4]. Vol. II, St. Louis, 1888 [Trans. Acad. Sci. St. Louis, vol. V, nos. 1 and 2].
HAWKINS, BENJ. A sketch of the Creek country, in 1798 and 99. Ga. Hist. Soc. Colls., vol. III, Savannah, 1848.
HITCHCOCK, GEN. E. A. Ms. Notes in possession of Mrs. W. H. Croffut, Washington, D. C.
HODGE, DAVID M. See Loughridge, R. M., and Hodge, David M.
HODGSON, ADAM. Remarks during a journey through North America in the years 1819, 1820, and 1821. New York, 1823.
JONES, C. C. History of Savannah, Ga., from its settlement to the close of the eighteenth century. Syracuse, N. Y., 1890.
LE MOYNE, JACQUES. Narrative of Le Moyne. Boston, 1875.
LE PAGE DU PRATZ, ANTOINE S. Histoire de la Louisiane. Tomes I–III. Paris, 1758. (Same, English trans., London, 1763, 1774.)
LOUGHRIDGE, R. M., and HODGE, DAVID M. English and Muskokee dictionary. St. Louis, 1890.
MACCAULEY, CLAY. The Seminole Indians of Florida. Fifth Ann. Rept. Bur. Ethn., pp. 469–531, Washington, 1887.
MERENESS, NEWTON, D., ed. Travels in the American Colonies. N. Y., 1916.
MILFORT [LE CLERC]. Mémoire ou coup-d'œil rapide sur mes différens voyages et mon séjour dans la nation Crĕck. Paris, 1802.
MOONEY, JAMES. Myths of the Cherokee. Nineteenth Ann. Rept. Bur. Amer. Ethn., pt. 1, Washington, 1900.
PICKETT, ALBERT J. History of Alabama, and incidentally of Georgia and Mississippi, from the earliest period. Vols. I–II. Charleston, 1851.
POPE, JOHN. Tour through the northern and western territories of the United States. Richmond, 1792.
SCHOOLCRAFT, HENRY R. Historical and statistical information respecting the history, condition and prospects of the Indian tribes of the United States. Parts I–VI. Phila., 1851–57.
SPECK, FRANK G. The Creek Indians of Taskigi town. Mem. Amer. Anthr. Asso., vol. II, pt. 2, Lancaster, Pa., 1907.
——— Ethnology of the Yuchi Indians. Anthr. Publs. Univ. Mus., Univ. Pa., vol. 1, no. 1, Phila., 1909.
STIGGINS, GEORGE. A historical narration of the genealogy, traditions, and downfall of the Ispocoga or Creek tribe of Indians writ by one of the tribe. (Ms. in possession of the Wisconsin Historical Society.)
TUGGLE, W. O. Myths of the Creeks. (Ms. in archives of Bur. Amer. Ethn.)

INDEX

Abihka: ceremonial title of, 614; one of four leading towns, 548

Achillea millefolium: medicinal use of, 663

Adams, Charlie: an informant, 528

adornment: for dance at busk, 600

Aesculus: medicinal use of, 658

ākitá dance: as a woman's dance, 528; described, 528; mention of, 524

Alabamas: belief of, in future life, 513; belief of, in supreme deity, 482; ceremony of, 544–45, 601–2; creation beliefs of, 487; dances of, described, 524–34; facial painting of, 524–25; ghost story of, 511–12; horned snake known to, 494; list of dances of, 524; medicines of, 663–66; name of, for deity, 482; relations of, with Hilibi, 568; sabía known to, 498; tales by, of supernatural beings, 498; use of cassine by, 542; witchcraft among, 634

Alindja: information furnished by, 546

alligator: association of, with disease, 647

alligator dance: described, 530; mention of, 524

angelica: medicinal use of, 657

animal dances: list of, 523–24; performance of, 610

animal spirits: animals' ability to talk attributed to, 489; association of, with disease, 638; diseases traced to, 638–39; propitiated by dances, 549; supernatural, 497–98

ant disease: symptoms of, 648

Antennaria: species of, medicinal use of, 668

Apalachicola: busk held at, 585

Arbeco Micco: mention of, 576

Aristolochia serpentaria: medicinal use of, 667

ark, sacred: a war medicine, 503

Arkansas Territory: Creek removal to, 505

Asclepias: species of, medicinal use of, 667, 668

Ascyrum: species of, medicinal use of, 666

Ascyrum multicaule: medicinal use of, 664

ási: as busk medicine, 547; ceremonial

drinking of, 538–44, 565, 604, 666; medicinal properties of, 666; mention of, 577, 582, 588, 598, 603, 606, 608; preparation of, 565; use of, 607 (*see also* black drink; cassine; *Ilex vomitoria*)

Asilanabi: mention of, 547; new fire ceremony of, 589

Atakapa: belief of, in chief deity, 482

atásá: as carried in women's dance, 549; as war symbol, 549

Atasi: at Tukabahchee busk, 559, 568

atcukliba: name of lizard, 495

aurora borealis: belief concerning, 479

badger: belief concerning, 644

ball for Creek game: supernatural object in, 492

ball game: at Tusgekee busk, 585

ball posts: ceremony of erecting, 544–45

Baptisia: medicinal use of, 658

bathing: as a purifying rite, 553, 601, 604; customs of, 520–21

bays: medicinal use of, 670

beans: celebration of new crop of, 550, 568

bear dance: described, 527; mention of, 523, 524

bear disease: description of, 640

bear's oil: use of, at busk, 598–99

beaver: illness caused by, 644

beaver dance: mention of, 523, 534

bed dance: mention of, 524; no details known of, 529

beds: erection of, for new ground, 545

Benzoin aestivale: medicinal use of, 657

Berryhill, William: dance described by, 527; informant, 534

Betula: medicinal use of, 659

Big Jack: Hilibi informant, 488; information from, 545, 546, 624

Bignonia crucigera: medicinal use of, 670

birch, white: medicinal use of, 659

birds: of prey, tabooed as food, 518; supernatural, 498

bison dance: described, 527; mention of, 523, 524; performance of, 573–74

bison disease: mention of, 640

bison hair: used as charm, 501

678 INDEX

McGillivray, Alexander: busk described by, 583–84

McKee, Mrs. James: information from, 666

malaria: remedy for, 655, 663

Malus: medicinal use of, 659

manitous of Algonkian tribes: comparison of spirits to, 511

"many snakes": meaning of the term, 644

many-snakes disease: 644

Master of Breath: mention of, 514, 584 (*see also* Hisagita imisi)

masters of waters: beliefs concerning, 490

"mastodon" disease: basis for name, 649

meat: burned in new fire, 605, 606

medical practices: influenced by whites, 622; methods of, 622–29 (*see also* diseases; doctors; medicines; priests)

medical treatment: result of failure of, 626; payment for, 623 (*see also* diseases; doctors; medicines)

medicine maker: office of, 620–21; power of, 621; selection of, 620

medicine mixers: duties of, 552

Medicine Spring Prairie OK: medicinal spring of, 669

medicines: buried under fire, 545; of the busk, 578, 607–8; ceremony of taking, 582; collection of, 552; composing the adiloga, 607; Creek, 639–63; making of, 563; precedence in taking, 558; preparation of, for busk, 569; religious significance of, 608; for stomp dance, 557; of the strong snake, 658; taken by fasters, 588; of the Tukabahchee, 509; used in ceremony, 552–53 (*see also* palladia; war physic)

Megillis Hadjo: beliefs concerning, 615; medical beliefs of, 644; prophet of Tukabahchee, 615; weather controlled by, 629–30

Meibomia: species of, medicinal use, 663

menstrual beliefs: 651

menstrual irregularity: remedies used for, 660, 662

meteors: belief concerning, 478

Mikasuki: dances known by, 524; dances of, 528, 530, 531, 533–34; medicines used by, 608; miko, stone under bed of, 545

miko hoyanīdja: a busk medicine, 547, 552; use of, 607, 617, 655

milkweed: medicinal use of, 667, 668

milky way: name given to, 513 (*see also* galaxy)

millepede disease: symptoms and treatment, 648

mistletoe: medicinal use of, 659

mole disease: symptoms of, 644

moles: belief concerning, 519

Monarda: species of, medicinal use of, 657

moon: beliefs concerning, 479–80; ceremonies timed by, 551, 553

Morning Star: Indian name for, 478

mortuary customs: 511, 513, 664 (*see also* burials; corpse; graves)

Morus rubra: medicinal use of, 659

mosquito dance: jokes played in, 534; mention of, 523

mulberry: connection of, with stomp dance, 550; French, medicinal use of, 663; medicinal use of, 659; sanctified by ceremony, 550

mullen: medicinal use of, 660–61

mumps: treatment of, 661, 668

music: accompanying dance, 600

musical instruments: 521–22, 628

Muskogees: hunting custom of, 516

muskrat: illness caused by, 644

Myrica: medicinal use of, 664

myths: creation, 487–88; illustrating diseases and remedies, 636–38

names: change of, for busk, 614; changed to cure sickness, 624

Nana Ishtohoollo: warning given by, 511

Natchez (Indians): belief of, concerning comets, 478; busk ceremonial of, 603; food of, eaten cold, 521; food taboos of 520–21; medicines of, 666–68; place of sun in worship of, 482; sabīa known to, 498

neuralgia: treatment of: 655

new corn crop: celebration of, 550, 568 (*see also* green corn dance; busk)

new fire: belief concerning, 594; burial under, of old fire, 589; distribution of, 555, 559, 563, 602, 603, 605; preparation for, 561; symbolic meaning of sticks of, 548 (*see also* busk fire)

new fire ceremony: 545, 555, 562–63, 570, 571–72, 577, 581, 583, 589, 595–96, 609

New Jersey tea: medicinal use of, 664

new year: celebrated by busk, 546, 551

Nokos īmała: information from, 655

Nokosi, Judge: mention of, 491

North Canadian River: mention of, 491

North Star: Indian name for, 478

Lightning Source UK Ltd.
Milton Keynes UK
UKHW042048101122
411892UK00016B/138